Leverage

Advance Praise

"Linda's experiences are relatable and validate that you are not alone in your struggle. She teaches you a foundational, whole-person approach to conquering your binge eating, which is often missing from traditional "diet and exercise" advice. For women open to a more holistic protocol, including calling upon their spirituality, I believe this book can help them to pursue a similar health transformation."

—Kathy Grassett
Certified Change and Wellness Coach

"So many people fail to connect their whole being with their binge eating issues. Linda gives straight forward, practical, and unique strategies that make the powerful holistic connection to once and for all overcome that obstacle, and to live a life you can be proud of!"

—Amanda Richards
Health and Fitness Coach

Leverage

The Guide to
End Your
Binge Eating

LINDA VANG

NEW YORK

LONDON • NASHVILLE • MELBOURNE • VANCOUVER

Leverage
The Guide to End Your Binge Eating

Published in New York, New York, by Morgan James Publishing in partnership with Difference Press. Morgan James is a trademark of Morgan James, LLC. www.MorganJamesPublishing.com

ISBN 978-1-64279-801-2 paperback
ISBN 978-1-64279-802-9 eBook
ISBN 978-1-64279-803-6 audio
Library of Congress Control Number: 2019913615

Cover Design by:
Christopher Kirk
www.GFSstudio.com

Interior Design by:
Bonnie Bushman
The Whole Caboodle Graphic Design

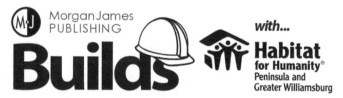

Morgan James is a proud partner of Habitat for Humanity Peninsula and Greater Williamsburg. Partners in building since 2006.

Get involved today! Visit
www.MorganJamesBuilds.com

This book is dedicated to my husband, Moua Xiong, of nine years (and beyond). Thank you for your continual support in everything I do. Thank you for supporting all my personal decisions for my own health journey. Your love and support do not go unnoticed.

Table of Contents

Foreword

In this candid book, Linda Vang unmasks the everyday challenges that face those affected by cycles of binge eating. Linda Vang not only connects with her readers through this emotional portrayal, but she also shares her secret to success. A path has been created for those suffering from food addiction, binge-eating cycles and those with an eating disorder. The only thing that readers must do is to take action and follow this road map to find their own success story. Many parts of this book spoke to me, despite not having the same struggles as Linda shares. One of my favorite quotes was when Linda states the following; "I learned that being pitiful and powerful takes the same amount of energy, so I could choose to be pitiful or powerful. I chose to be powerful." Linda guides the reader through a process of taking their power back and taking control of both their internal and external world in order to reflect their best selves.

The myriad of daily choices amidst a busy, stressful lifestyle can leave us grasping for ways to cope and manage our stress. The ability to become mindful, engage in a deep internal process of healing emotional, spiritually and physically has been laid out by Linda in beautiful simplicity. Linda's own journey of healing proves that becoming healthy and changing our lifestyles to reflect our own self-worth is not only probable, but also possible with the tools laid out in this book. Linda Vang started this journey many years ago as my student and it is wonderfully fulfilling to see her becoming my teacher. Thank you, Linda Vang for sharing your story to empower others to live theirs.

Megan E. Van Zyl PhD Hon, MA, NTP
Your Cancer Expert
www.cancerpeaceuniversity.com

Disclaimer

The author of this book is not a physician. The author is not offering any medical advice. If you are in need of medical advice, please reach out to a medical doctor. The author is not prescribing the use of any of the concepts and techniques mentioned in this book without the consent of a doctor. The purpose of this book is for educational and informational use only. This book is not a substitute for medical advice or treatment from specific medical conditions or disorders. The author does not agree to diagnose or treat any disease or condition. If you choose to use the concepts and techniques discussed in this book, the author assumes no responsibility for your actions.

Introduction

You are at your wit's end with this never-ending cycle of binge eating. As much as you want to completely avoid thinking about taking control of your binge eating, it just seems impossible. It's impossible because binge eating has consumed every inch of you and has affected every area of your life. What used to seem like only a physical struggle is starting to affect you mentally and emotionally, and has caused you to lose your self-esteem and self-control. You cry every other day, and you can't find the motivation to remain focus anymore. Your life is slowly spiraling out of control.

Despite wanting to give up and just stay in bed all day, you somehow find yourself up, getting ready for another day in motion just to do what you need to get done. You are hopeful that today will be the day you finally break free from your binge eating habit. But unfortunately, even more than hopeful, you are doubtful. Doubt takes over because you are afraid you may never be able to be in control of your binge eating cycles. You have been through this cycle before, where your first three to four hours are spent being positive and hopeful, the next few hours are spent talking yourself out of a healthy lifestyle, and your hours right before bed are spent feeling sorry for yourself, frustrated, and worthless because once again you have failed to take control and feel like you have hit rock bottom.

Just Another Day of Broken Promises

You are probably telling yourself right now that today is just another day, another day of giving in to binge eating. Everything seems quite hopeless right now. You are so used to your cycle of broken promises. You continue to tell yourself that today, tomorrow, next week, or next year will be the year you will finally be in control of your binge eating habit. Your never-ending binge eating cycle seems to be such a part of you now that, once lunchtime rolls around every day, without thinking, the right thing to do seems to be to break the goal you had in mind to eat healthier and eat whatever your heart desires.

Even though you wake up feeling refreshed and ready to conquer this habit of yours, by the time lunchtime comes, you seem to have forgotten all the promises you made to yourself just this morning. Only once the damage is done, and you have eaten everything in sight are you reminded of how your life is really spiraling out of control. Not only is your eating habit out of control, but your personal relationships also seem to be falling apart, and your love life seems to be dead. Your professional life—the only thing that once was your motivation and the one thing you have worked so hard for—seems to have also come to a halt. You are screaming for help, but no one, including God, seems to hear you. You can't focus at work, and you find yourself only going through the motions to get through the day with absolutely no motivation. It seriously is a never-ending cycle that is completely draining you out.

Trust and believe, I know you are here for a reason. You are here because not only are you frustrated, but you still have a little more hope left in you. I want to take some time to praise you because even though you may feel as though you are here as your last resort, it shows me that you are willing to give it one more try. I hope this book gives you the inspiration you need to understand that your life and your health are worth one more try.

This Cycle Has No Ending

It's Sunday night. You finally got the chance to relax after a busy weekend spent catching up with friends and family. Of course, none of those gatherings lacked any food. In fact, they were filled with lots of junk foods, fried foods, and so many options of meat to choose from. You spent two full days mindlessly eating. You came home from each gathering and went to sleep, starting on Friday, feeling extremely full.

You are finally sitting comfortably on your couch mentally preparing yourself for the upcoming week. You first go through work and mentally go through your to-do list for the week. You finally get to reflect and focus on yourself and your personal goals. You know that, once again, you broke your promise to yourself about finally getting it together and taking control of your binge eating habit. You take some time to remind yourself that it's Monday, and tomorrow starts a new day, which means a new start to a healthier, sexier you. You got this! You even took some time today to prepare your breakfast and lunch for tomorrow. You are finally going to be committed and succeed in living a healthier lifestyle. You remind yourself that you have a birthday coming up and there just isn't any way you are going be feeling disgusted and looking bulgy and bloated this year. You are so tired of looking and feeling unhealthy every day, let alone looking horrible at your next birthday celebration. This is it—good-bye to the old you!

Monday comes and you are feeling good. Totally pumped. You even got in a good stretch this morning. You woke up just a little bit earlier to make sure you don't feel rushed. You are feeling even better on your way to work because you pumped yourself up for the day by listening to nothing but feel-good music. You get to work, and everything seems to start out great. As you work through your morning, you start to get more and more client complaints. You can't seem to get anything done because you are so busy dealing with customer's complaints. You still continue holding on to your dreams and hopes of finally controlling your binge eating habit. You take two seconds to eat what you packed for breakfast. Lunchtime rolls around. Just as you start to take your home-cooked meal out, your two close co-workers ask if you would like to join them at the burger joint a few blocks down. Without thinking, you agree to go. On the walk there, you mentally promise yourself that you will only eat a salad, and at most fries, if you really need to give in to your temptations. You get to lunch and realize that your co-workers are getting the usual loaded burgers and fries. You start to give in a little, talking yourself out of eating healthy. You continue to browse the menu for something healthier. Healthier just doesn't seem appetizing to you. You have convinced yourself that you will give yourself just one more day to cheat. You can start tomorrow. Besides, you have forty-one more days just before your birthday. Forty-one days should give you enough time to at least lose five to ten pounds. Before you know it, you are ordering burgers and fries. Once you are done with your burgers and fries, you remind yourself that, since you have already broken your diet, you might as well go all out and get yourself a dessert, and even a meal to-go for tonight's dinner because you know you are going to be too lazy after work to cook.

You spend the rest of the day feeling sluggish at work. You can't concentrate or focus. You would just prefer to take a nice nap. You also spend the rest of the day mentally beating yourself up for cheating. You realize that the cycle of binge eating will never be broken. Nothing seems to be going the way you hoped.

You get home and don't feel good at all. Your stomach pain and other physical symptoms seem to have progressed. You get home and finally get one moment to yourself. You express your day of failure to your significant other. He just doesn't seem to get your struggle. Instead of just hearing you out, he decides he wants to give you advice that you actually do not want at the moment. All you want to do is to run to your room and cry out your frustrations. But instead, you get distracted with your favorite reality show that you have been looking forward to watching all day.

You end the night more than devastated with yourself for breaking your promise, but continue to promise yourself that tomorrow will be better.

Don't Give Up On Me

I have been exactly where you currently are. I know you are feeling so stressed out right now, you are at your wit's end. Even though you just want to give up, you realize that if you do not take control of your health now, everything else in your life will come crashing down at a faster rate than you can even imagine. Even accomplishments in your life that once seemed successful, and goals you have worked so hard for will also start to crash. Even if you can find the motivation to get up every day and just simply go through the motions in life, with your progressing physical symptoms, you realize that one day your health will deteriorate, which will lead to chronic, life-long illnesses.

Once your body deteriorates, you will truly feel worthless. You would have absolutely no more confidence and no self-esteem left, not that there is anything left at the moment. Your emotions will go flying out the window. You will probably be crying every second of the day; it's already bad enough you are crying at least every other day now. Your parents, especially your mom, would definitely think and act upon her thoughts, expressing to you even more that you have become the person she knew you always were, a person who would never do anything significant with her life.

You Got This!

Don't worry. Trust and believe that you have this book in your hand at the right moment. Even though it might feel like it's too late for you, it's not. Magic happens when you hit rock bottom. Once you hit rock bottom, giving it your all is your only option. If it means you have to try just one more time, you will find the strength to do so, even when you feel like giving up.

You got this! Soon, you are going to start each day feeling pumped and refreshed, and end your day feeling even more motivated for tomorrow. You will see that taking it one day at a time becomes easier and even a bit fun as you start to see improvements in your mind, body, and spirit.

Your body will appreciate your healthier lifestyle and unexpected surge of energy. Your body can only give you back what you give it. When you give your body love, it gives you love with a boost of confidence. When you give your body fuel, it gives you energy. When you give your body emotional relief, it gives you happiness and joy. What will you be giving your body?

Just One More Step

In order for anything to truly work, it starts with trusting the process, even if you don't completely understand the process. It starts with taking one step at a time in the right direction, and believing that God has your back and will continue to lead you in the right direction. If you keep going, the process only gets easier.

I want you to take a moment to just soak in how it will feel if you just take one more step forward in the right direction.

It's Sunday night. You finally got the chance to relax after a busy weekend spent catching up with friends and family. Of course, none of those gatherings lacked any food. In fact, they were filled with lots of junk foods, fried foods, and so many options of meat to choose from. You are so proud of yourself that you did not spend your whole weekend mindlessly eating. Before you headed out to each gathering, you fueled your body with real nutritious food that would keep you filled up for most of the day. You even packed a little food to remind yourself that you have a healthier option available, if needed. That small piece of cake you did decide to indulge in felt more fulfilling than your usual mindless eating. Better yet, even two of your friends complimented you on how your face suddenly has this nice glow to it.

You are finally sitting comfortably on your couch, mentally preparing yourself for the upcoming week. You finally get to reflect and focus on yourself and your personal goals. You review how successful your first binge-free week has been. It was a bit challenging, but you survived. Even though you had one cheat meal, it was much better than a cycle of broken promises. You take some time to remind yourself that it's Monday, and tomorrow starts a new day, which means a new start. You got this! You can't wait to see what this week brings you as you keep going. You remind yourself that you have a birthday coming up, and this is finally the year you will be looking and feeling good. You are more determined to keep going. You have come so far. It's time to say good-bye to the old you!

Monday comes and you are feeling good. You grab your breakfast and lunch you have prepared for the day. You are feeling pumped. You get to work, and everything seems to start out great. As you work through your morning, you start to get more and more client complaints. You can't seem to get anything done because you are so busy dealing with customer's complaints. You remind yourself that no matter how stressful work becomes, you have come too far to give in to your usual cravings when you are faced with stress at work. Bring it on, stress! Lunchtime rolls around. Just as you start to take your home-cooked meal out, your two close co-workers ask if you would like to join them at the burger joint a few blocks down. You are tempted to join them just for a salad, but you realize what happened the last time you promised yourself a salad. You decide to let them know that you brought your own lunch and will join them next time. They walk out of your office telling you how proud of you for sticking to a healthier lifestyle they are. You remind your coworkers that you have forty-one more days just before your birthday. Forty-one days should give you enough time to at least lose ten to fifteen pounds. You are looking forward to feeling great and looking good.

You spend the rest of the day feeling energized at work. Your focus is great, and you just can't wait to go home to go check out the gym that you just finally got around to signing up to join. You spend the rest of the day giving yourself a pat on the back for not giving in. Everything seems to be progressing just fine.

You get home and you feel good. Your stomach pain and other physical symptoms seem to have slowly disappeared. You get home and finally get one moment to yourself. You express your successful day to your significant other. Instead of giving you his usual advice that you don't even want to hear, he tells you how proud he is of you and your progress. All you want to do at this moment is enjoy this feeling of accomplishment. Before you head out to the gym, you and your significant other decided to cook a homemade meal and enjoy it together.

You end the night in delight. You often find yourself smiling. You are glad to know that you will finally keep your promises of continuing this journey when tomorrow comes.

Conquering Your Fears

I know how you are feeling. I know you are wondering if this process will actually work for you. You have gone through so many protocols that seem to work for everyone else, except you. I can't promise you this process will be easy because it is a lifestyle change, but I can promise that I will give you the best resources and tools to help leverage your binge eating habit. I will also hold your hand through every step and make sure each step is as easy to comprehend as possible.

You are probably wondering where you should start because you hate being loaded with so much information that you will probably never put to use. There will be a lot of information. You are to follow each step and concept exactly how it is written. You should practice and implement each concept and technique you learn as soon as possible but while going through each exercise you should not rush yourself, and take as much time as you need.

As you begin using these concepts and techniques, you will even wonder if you have enough time for this. Of course you do! We are talking about your life and your health. If you can spend eight-plus hours at work, your life and health are worth at least a few hours of your day. The most you will have to do is squeeze in an extra thirty minutes to an hour to complete all the techniques I will be teaching you.

I know that the lingering fear of failing you may have is because you have had this binge eating cycle for so long. Success just seems so far away. One step at a time, one day at a time is all I am asking from you. So what if you do sneak in a cheat meal? You will be completely fine; all you need to do is get right back on track! Get back on track with your next meal, not the next day because, as we know, too many times before tomorrow may bring broken promises. The best time to start is now, at your next your meal, even if you messed up. The only way this protocol will not work is if you give up trying these steps. These steps will be life-changing, and if you keep up with them, they will be everlasting.

Being Prepared For the Storm Ahead

Your journey ahead, like any worthwhile journey, will be tough. There are days you might feel like you are soaring, and no one can stop you from reaching your goals. But there will be days where you just feel like, regardless of your progress so far, you just want to give up.

In this book, I will equip you with all the resources and information you need to make those hard days a bit easier. I am going to show you step-by-step, chapter by chapter how to build yourself a strong foundation for those days you want to give in and give up. You will be prepared for the storm ahead. Soon, your temptations and cravings will be part of your past, but just in case they pop up once in a while, you will be well prepared to tackle them.

Some of the concepts and techniques will be new to you. I will give you a new perspective and a new healing experience. You might even think it's a bit weird, but the best way to tackle this and your binge eating habit is head on. It's worth experiencing and trying things you have not yet tried because what you have been trying most of your life has not yet worked.

I Got You!

In this book, I will show you how you can use these simple concepts to create a life free of binge eating. You will even learn to create the life you have always wanted beyond binge eating.

I am here to remind you that no matter what you do, giving up is not an option. When you feel like giving up, I want you to think back to the day when you cried your heart out because you did not get the dream job you wanted after you graduated college. Did you give up? No. You kept pushing forward. Look at how successful you are now. Keep in mind, everything happens for a reason.

I am going to be that coach that keeps pushing you to reach just a little higher than you believe you can. I am going to show you that you got this, and I got you! I am going to be here to keep pushing you forward, to keep letting you know that you are worth one more try, that your success story is worth passing on, and hopefully one day, you will choose to make a difference in both your life and the lives of others.

Stay tuned, there's more to come! Are you ready?! Let's get started!

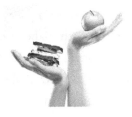

Chapter 1

I Learned How to Swim in Deep Waters Because I Could Not Afford to Drown

Trust me when I say I understand the problem you are currently struggling with. I have been in your shoes and am still actively engaging in a healthier lifestyle. I am proof that as long as you don't give up, and you continue to strive for better, you, too, can overcome your binge eating habit. For years, I had to deal with my own binge eating habit. My life and health seemed to have spiraled out of control right before my eyes. Before I knew it, my binge eating habit created the life I never wanted. I never wanted to become unhealthy or be diagnosed with type 2 diabetes. I grew up seeing my father going in and out of hospitals and struggling with all the other health complications that came with diabetes, and that was the last route I would have wanted for myself.

When I was diagnosed with diabetes at the age of twenty-eight, I was devasted. As if struggling with binge eating was not enough, now I also had to deal with diabetes. My binge eating habits and unhealthy lifestyle caused me to hit rock bottom. I felt like I was drowning. However, looking back, this was definitely my wake-up call. I knew that I could not afford to give up and drown. On a brighter note, diabetes has helped me to take control of my binge eating habits and has made me become more aware of what I am putting in my mouth. Even though it was a very tough journey, diabetes gave me the opportunity to be able to take care of my body as a young adult. I am glad I was not hit with diabetes at a later time in my life because it would be harder for me both emotionally and mentally, and much harder for my body to heal.

Here is my story, and I hope that it will inspire you. I hope that you will come to understand that controlling your binge eating habit is possible—yes, even for you.

A Whole New World

If you are anything like me, lifestyle changes in the form of nutrition and healthy eating has been by far the toughest. Learning to love myself by treating this temple of mine better has proved to be extremely challenging. When I started living a healthier lifestyle, I stepped into new and unknown territory and was terrified to learn that I would have to completely change the way I ate. I would later find out that I even had to change the way I thought about food.

I have seen many health experts quickly change their lives around, going from a previous 350-pound person to someone that is now lean and fit. I continue to wonder why my nutritional journey didn't come as easy and as natural as these experts made it seem. For a very, very long time, I was frustrated and disappointed in myself because even when I became a health coach, I had every resource at the tip of my hand and I knew all that I needed to know in terms of nutrition in order to heal, but still nothing seemed to work. I had to learn the hard way that knowing and doing were two totally different things.

Of course, I should have known this lifestyle change was not going to be easy. Even though I wanted to and should have jumped into this new healthy lifestyle full force, I didn't.

I grew up with eating habits that were far from healthy. I learned later that my body can only heal if I give it the chance to heal by making a lot of dietary changes. I grew up, for the most part, in a very happy home. There was never a dull moment with a family of nine siblings and both parents. Even though we were poor, my parents made sure we were fed. My mom made sure to teach us her very best when it came to cooking our own food. She wanted me to be independent and prepare me to later be a proper wife.

My family and I ate mostly Asian dishes. If we were not eating a homecooked Asian meal, I ate processed foods or foods that were convenient, such as hot dogs, eggs, and noodles. By age seven, I already knew how to cook very basic foods, which included frying my own eggs, frying or boiling my own hot dogs, and making my own noodles. By the age of fourteen, I learned how to cook more intricate meals, such as chicken curry. During the weekdays, because there were so many of us and my parents were so busy with life and trying to make a living, I remember eating processed and unhealthy foods, which my mother taught me how to cook at a young age, along with the rice that was made either by my mother or older siblings.

Yes, of course, we had homemade and naturally prepared meals and often ate around the table whenever my parents had the time to cook; this was usually the weekends. I thoroughly enjoyed the many meals spent eating with the whole family. It was a time to catch up, laugh, and even disagree a bit with my siblings. Some of these meals consisted of boiled chicken, stir-fry, and vegetable soup with or without meat, along with, at least for me, a lot of rice. Even nowadays, my family still makes jokes about me and my love for rice. I do really love white rice!

Rice was a staple food for me, as it is for many Asian families. But for me, even as a young child, because there were so many of us and food seemed to be limited, I learned to love rice and overeat rice at each meal. I remember, as I sat around the dining table, I thought to myself too many times that if I did not hurry up and eat, I would struggle to get a second serving or go without one because there were simply too many of us for everyone to get a second serving. I learned that even if I did not get a second serving, rice would always fill me up, because of course we always had plenty of it. I later learned that those extra servings of rice that tasted so delicious with my noodles, eggs, and hot dogs were detrimental to my health. I eventually had to learn to reduce and periodically eliminate rice from my diet.

Growing up in such a close-knit family, we would often spend most of our weekends with both immediate and extended family. Of course, this meant more food! These gatherings were filled with laughter and memories, but most of all an abundance of food—mostly homecooked food filled with not exactly the healthiest ingredients. This would pose an even a bigger challenge for me. Imagine having a big Christmas dinner almost every weekend or every other weekend.

I was always a heavier-set person. I started noticing my body was a bit different from most of my female classmates during high school. When everyone was decently in good shape, I felt like I was the only one out of shape. I noticed that my menstrual cycles were nothing close to normal, like my female classmates. My menstrual cycle came when it wanted, if it came at all. I would get my menstrual cycle only about once or twice a year. I went to my high school nurse to see if I could get advice on how I could get my wacky hormones in control and back into balance. Without even running any lab work or diagnosing what it was that caused my hormonal imbalances, she was quick to advise that I get on birth control to regulate my menstrual cycles. Little did I know, birth control was detrimental to my health. I would later learn that birth control did nothing more than mask my symptoms by forcing my menstrual cycle to show up every month. Birth control only caused more disruption to my already imbalanced hormones because it kept my estrogen at a continually high level, which is not normal and can possibly lead to other health issues, like gallbladder or liver complications, increased risk of blood clot, heart attacks, or strokes.

Through these occasional visits to my school nurse, I also found out that because of my elevated glucose levels, I was considered pre-diabetic. I was informed that there was nothing they could do to help me with my elevated glucose levels until I was actually diagnosed as a diabetic. Unfortunately, in 2014, I was actually diagnosed as a diabetic. I was informed that I would need to be on medication as soon as possible. I was also informed that I would be on medication for the rest of my life, and that was the only and the best way I could manage my diabetes.

Even as a young high school student, I knew something was off. My gut feeling knew that being told there was nothing I could do as a pre-diabetic to prevent becoming diabetic was off. As a young adult, I was always trained to trust my doctors, and that was exactly what I did. I even somehow managed to believe that if there was nothing I could do to prevent diabetes, I could eat whatever I wanted and as much as I wanted. I wish I had done more research before I was actually diagnosed with diabetes. Unfortunately, I didn't know any better and was way too busy with school to even care about my health at the time. I didn't know where to start and there was just too much information out there. I could find anything I wanted on Google. The hardest part for me was sorting out all the conflicting information that was out there. I didn't know what was actually best for me. I would find different sources of information that stated a vegetable only diet was good for me and other sources informed me that limiting my carbohydrates, including most fruits and vegetables was best.

All I knew was that I was stuck with being a pre-diabetic (and later a diabetic), and that was the sad, uneducated information my own trusted high school nurse gave me.

Each Mistake Is a Lesson

My health journey has not always been an easy one. It is still something I am working to improve every day. I have come a long way and am no longer held down by binge eating, but temptations will always find a way to creep up on me. I am actually hit with temptations weekly, if not daily. But I am definitely doing a better job of learning from the mistakes I made along the way and hope that you will also learn from my mistakes. Take some time to reflect upon my mistakes and try not to make the same mistakes I made, which will make your journey much easier.

My first mistake was keeping myself too busy with school and work. I worked so hard to excel in my career that I completely neglected my health. My career caused me unnecessary stress. I stayed late at work and stayed up thinking about it. I didn't give myself any time to eat or cook the proper food I needed to fuel my body. I didn't want to make time for any physical activity. When I did have time, I would be too exhausted to want to do anything else but eat myself some good tasting fried food in front of the TV while watching my reality shows. Don't overwork yourself for things that are not everlasting. Money will come and go. Do not slave and lose yourself trying to earn yourself some money.

My never-ending binge eating cycle continued over and over because I talked myself into thinking that, eventually, I would land on or find the perfect day to start my healthier lifestyle. I even convinced myself that Mondays are better than Tuesdays to start my healthy lifestyle and that even days are better than odd days. I lied to myself that tomorrow, next week, or next year would be the perfect day to start my healthier lifestyle. Instead of focusing on my next healthy meal, I always started with the tomorrows that didn't really come—or maybe it came, but I never really committed to tomorrow like I said I would because I knew I would get another tomorrow to try again.

With so much information available, I had no idea where to start. I made the huge mistake of not turning to all of nature's goodness, like vegetables and fruits. Instead, I focused on unimportant things like calorie counting or paying attention to the numbers on the scale and weighing myself way too often. I found myself in the middle of too many fad diets that did not work, were too boring to follow, or left me hungry all the time. All it did was create my desire to have a binge eating session. When in doubt, turn to nature.

The hardest mistake for me to understand was discovering that I was unique and there was no "one size fits all" diet plan or fad diet I could follow to accomplish my nutritional goals. I always wanted the body other people had. I had to learn that my body is different, it may react differently, it may take longer to heal or longer to see and feel any difference. The foods that fuel others may not be fuel to my body. The foods that fulfilled others may not be fulfilling to me. I had to learn how to be patient with myself and my results, and had to realize that being consistent would help me accomplish my goals.

The biggest mistake I made, due to a lack of knowledge, was that I didn't have a strong enough foundation. I didn't understand that I was a whole being. A being that not only existed as a physical body, but also had a mind and spirit. I focused way too much on my physical being and my physical results. This probably did more harm than good. It was only later that I learned I needed to leverage my healing and binge eating with concepts and techniques that would support my mind, body, and spirit.

The Perfection of God's Timing and Resources

I look back at my journey and realize just how crazy it is that the Lord has set me up so perfectly in preparation for this journey, something only the Lord can do and control. After I was diagnosed with diabetes, I decided to enroll and get my health coaching certificate so that I could make a difference in the lives I touched. Similar to finishing any kind of certificate or degree, you are left to figure out on your own how you want to best use your knowledge gained.

While I was in the process of completing my health coaching program, one of my health coaching colleagues introduced me to a Nutritional Therapy Practitioner (NTP), someone she had only met briefly at a local health foods grocery store. This NTP, now a great mentor of mine, had a training program that was currently enrolling students. Her program sounded amazing; it was something I could not miss out on. For some reason, I knew it would be amazing knowledge I would be missing out on if I did not sign up for her program. My gut feeling was right. I learned so much from this amazing woman. She has taught me so many nutritional skills and so much knowledge that I have used to get over my own binge eating and helped clients. Better yet, get this—she was the one who reintroduced me to the Lord. How good the Lord is to already have prepared me for this journey. Can you just take a moment to imagine what the Lord has already prepared for you on your journey?

Strive to Be a Blessing to Others

I completed a health coaching certificate knowing that I wanted to make a difference in the lives of people I come in contact with. I wanted to see people excel in life even if they were unfortunately hit with a health crisis. I wanted to let people, just like you, know that even if the doctor tells you that you cannot do anything to change the state of your health, you certainly can. I want to be the mentor that I never had in high school, who could have prevented me from being diagnosed with diabetes. I want to make life easier for people, just like you, so you can skip over all the trials and errors I had to go through and skip having to shuffle through all the conflicting information out there.

Regardless of your broken promises to yourself, the binge eating cycles that seem to never end, and the frustrations, I am here to tell you it is possible. You can do it! One day, just like me, you will be able to use your own struggles and story to help and bless others in need. I wasn't even sure how I was going to make an impact in people's lives, but now I am certain my own health journey will be the stepping stone for my life's mission and the purpose that the Lord has for me.

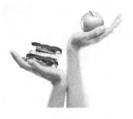

Chapter 2

Diving Deep

The truth is, successfully conquering your binge eating habit is more than just nutrition. It's about the emotions that come up, it's about the willpower that doesn't seem to work when you need it most, and it's about those many times you're wondering where God is when you need Him most.

In this book, I will discuss the concepts and foundations you need in place to successfully conquer any temptations that may come up. I will teach you how to successfully implement these concepts in your everyday lives. You are going to learn more than just how nutrition can help you avoid binge eating. In fact, you are going to learn how to use your mind, emotions, and relationship with God to leverage yourself in order to control your binge eating.

More Than Just Knowing

The problem with a lot of the information that teaches you how to free yourself from binge eating is that all they do is focus solely on food and nutrition. They expect that once you know everything you need to know about how, when, and what to eat, you are well on your way to starting a new lifestyle that is free from binge eating. Like I have learned, knowing and doing are two totally different things. You can have all the resources readily available to you, but if you are not given any information on how to set yourself up for success and how to tackle temptations and cravings, you ultimately end up setting yourself up to fail. Most of the information out there doesn't think about the actual struggle you face when implementing their protocol. They don't think about your failed willpower and the challenges you face. They don't take into consideration that you are a whole being with a mind, body, and spirit.

In this book, I will approach binge eating much differently than what you are probably used to. We are going to build for you a strong foundation, taking into consideration that sometimes willpower alone just isn't enough, and that you are whole, with a mind, body, and spirit. This means that all aspects of your life have the ability to affect you physically and affect your never-ending binge eating cycles. The ideas and techniques I will teach you will help you leverage yourself and your binge eating cycles so that when you do dive into the nutritional part of the book, you should have discovered and experienced so much about what is holding you back that tackling the actual nutrition part becomes a breeze.

In each chapter, I will discuss concepts and techniques for you to implement so that you will be able to leverage your binge eating. I will go into great details about using the energy (quantum physics) that surrounds you, using the relationship you have with the Lord, discovering emotional healing to build yourself a new slate and emotional stability in order to tackle binge eating, ensuring the whole process feels less complicated and frustrating. I suggest spending seven to ten days in each chapter, exploring and implementing the concepts and techniques in each chapter. Keep in mind the goal is to spend as much time as you need in each chapter, this will allow you to experience how using quantum physics, building your relationship with God, and emotional healing can help you if you continue to use it daily.

Let's quickly dive into how leveraging different aspects of your life can help you finally take control of your binge eating cycles. When I was battling my own binge eating habits, the definition of leverage I kept in mind was, "The ability to influence a system, or an environment, in a way that multiplies the outcome of one's efforts without a corresponding increase in the consumption of resources. In other words, leverage is the advantageous condition of having a relatively small amount of cost yield a relatively high level of returns." To me, this meant that, in order to take control of my eating habit, I was going to have to invest some time in myself and act upon these exact concepts and techniques that I will be teaching you. I learned that the positive changes I started to see in my life outweighed the small amount of time, effort, and energy I spent in order to achieve the life I always wanted. As you start to see these positive changes in your own life, trust me, you will naturally want to continue to invest more time and resources in yourself because these positive changes will impact all areas of your life.

These techniques and concepts will become an important part of your life as you set yourself free from binge eating. My goal is to teach you how to work smarter and not harder towards your binge-free life. Working smarter means implementing a daily routine that is enjoyable and effective. You will see how simply adding thirty minutes to one hour into your daily schedule will drastically change your life. You will start to gain more energy, more focus, and even rid yourself of your physical symptoms.

Can You Find Success in Your Daily Habits?

"The secret to success is found in your daily habit."
–Unknown

Did you know that a highly successful person can observe what you do in only one day and be able to determine if you will be successful? That's right. In only one day! You know why? This is because your success is found in your daily habits; in the things you do daily. Not in a huge event that takes months or even years to plan, but in your daily habits. So how will you succeed at freeing yourself from binge eating? You guessed it! Implementing these concepts and techniques you learn right into your daily lives. It might take waking up thirty minutes to an hour earlier than usual or going to sleep one hour later than usual, but that one hour extra, trust me, it will be life-changing!

The goal is to create a daily routine that is thirty minutes to an hour long. You can choose whether you want to implement this daily routine in the morning as the first thing you do right after you wake up, or you can choose to implement this in the evening as you wind down for the night. I was never a morning person and completed my daily routine during the evenings for a very long time. I finally decided recently to try adjusting my sleep schedule to incorporate my daily routine into my morning instead. I stuck with my morning routine because it just seems to get me more energized for the day, set my tone for the day, and even help me mentally set my goals for the day. I have included a sample of what my morning routine and daily routine look like to help you create a daily routine that will work for you (see Appendix A).

Even though the concepts introduced in this book go into great detail, implementing the techniques actually do not take too long. I made sure the techniques I shared with you in this book are easy to implement into your daily routine. I understand how important it is to have a routine that is simple and easy to implement because I am the type who could never commit to implementing processes and techniques that are too long and complicated. Once you get the hang of how you can use these concepts and techniques to leverage your binge eating habit, you can change things up and be as creative as you want. Make the process unique, fun, and enjoyable according to your own needs and goals.

A Quick Dive

Below, I will introduce to you a quick summary of the concepts and techniques that you can implement into your daily lives to help support you in controlling your binge eating. Don't worry about how to use them yet; you will learn everything you need to know about them in the following chapters. Some of these ideas may be new and totally different to you. As for now, all you have to do is soak them in.

You will:

- Understand what quantum physics is and how you can use this knowledge to incorporate daily meditation to create the life you want, which includes freeing yourself from your binge eating cycle. You will learn how to create a new state of being for yourself, break free from allowing your body to control your mind which has caused these binge eating cycles, and eventually learn how to let your body embrace this new guilt-free, binge-free, healthier you.

- Learn how to develop a relationship with God that will help you understand who you are, renew your mind, and understand what is holding you back from successfully breaking free of your binge eating habit.

- Learn how negative memory and trauma have impacted you emotionally. Understand how these negative emotions may have been draining you and holding you back from reaching your goals. You will discover how to release these negative emotions in order to create emotional stability in your life.

- Learn to create an environment for yourself both at home and at work that will help support your healthier lifestyle.
- Finally, after creating a successful foundation for yourself, you will learn all that you need to know nutritionally. I will go into what you should eat, and what you should not eat.

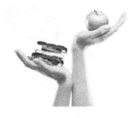

Chapter 3

Quantum Physics

*B*elieve it or not, you have experienced quantum physics in your life. I would go as far as to say even in your daily life. Even if you are not aware of it, quantum physics is a part of us. Have you ever met someone and you both instantly connected? That is quantum physics working. It is your energy aligning with each other that creates such instant connections. Quantum physics is used in our everyday lives, allowing microwaves, x-rays, and MRI scans to properly work.

Quantum physics is definitely more complicated than just aligning energy, but for the sake of our purpose and to help you overcome binge eating, I am going to give you a very simple explanation of what quantum physics is so you can learn and understand the concept in order to use it intentionally in your everyday life. Once you have learned how to integrate quantum physics into your life, taking control of binge eating can become a lot less stressful and complicated. Besides, if you are anything like me, science just isn't my thing, but learning how to use it to change my eating habit and lifestyle has been nothing short of amazing.

What Is Quantum Physics, and How Does It Affect Me?

If you think back to your high school science class, you probably remember learning the concept of atoms. Quantum physics states that all matter, in its smallest unit of matter, exists as atoms, and even smaller, matter exists as subatomic particles that make up an atom. These subatomic particles exist as an invisible field of energy. These subatomic particles and energies exist as pure potential and possibilities and can only come to life when we observe them. You and I are also made up of atoms and subatomic particles in our smallest units. This ultimately means that you and I, including our conscious minds, exist as energy. As energy, we all have the ability to communicate with each other. By observing and communicating with energy, we have the ability to influence our physical realities.

I know what you are thinking. "What exactly do you mean, 'observe subatomic particles and energy?' Didn't you just tell me subatomic particles are invisible? So how is it that I can observe energy that is invisible?" You can absolutely observe energy. Let me explain. You observe and communicate with energy through your thoughts and feelings. This means that energy is pretty much nothing unless you communicate with it. When you communicate with the energy that exists as potential, you are able to manifest what you choose to observe into your physical world. You can manifest good and bad physical realities. When you are constantly communicating with the energy around you that you are fat, ugly, and worthless, that is exactly what will continue to manifest into your physical reality. Once you can start communicating that you are in control, beautiful, and energetic, that is what you will get in return. Communication is key. My guess is, like myself for many years, you have been manifesting your broken promises and the life you have been wanting to break away from. You have unknowingly been using the negative beliefs you have about yourself and your never-ending binge eating cycle to create exactly what you have been trying to get away from. If done correctly, you can also manifest your desired reality. You will learn how to create positive new thoughts and feelings that will help you to reach your goals and live a better version of yourself. Your future outcomes really are in your own hands.

Imagine this: you get up every morning. You start your day on a positive note, hoping that today will finally be the day you stop binge eating. You even go as far as to think about finally getting around to accomplishing everything you have always wanted to accomplish once you can finally control your binge eating and achieve the body you have always wanted. That is, until your lunch hour comes around and food starts calling your name and your hunger pains are unbearable. You finally give in after trying to be on your best behavior. The binge eating cycle starts all over again. You not only eat anything and everything you see, but you stuff in as much as you can. By the time you realize what just happened, you start to feel horrible and disgusted with what you just did, and your mind starts racing. You start to tell yourself, "Who cares? I already ruined the start to my healthier lifestyle. I'm going to eat whatever and whenever I want because this is going to be my last day of eating horribly, and I can start tomorrow."

But of course, it doesn't end there. Once you are stuffed and the damage is done, you start to beat yourself up. You tell yourself you are fat and ugly, that you worthless, and that you will always be a failure. You even start to feel like breaking your binge eating habit is impossible. You see, this is exactly what you communicated to the quantum realm. Remember, the quantum realm is energy full of potential and possibility. It is waiting to fulfill your command. You continue to create a cycle of binge eating because you continue to communicate to the world that you are fat and ugly, you will always be a failure and breaking your binge eating habit is impossible. This is exactly what the quantum realm has manifested into your physical world because of your own observation.

Don't be discouraged. What I am telling you is that you can use quantum physics to both manifest the life you want, no longer controlled by binge eating, and also use quantum physics to help make the process of breaking your binge eating habit less frustrating. This is going to be a life-long process. Nothing good comes easily, and you should not expect changes overnight. I will give you the tools and share my experiences of how I have used quantum physics to break myself from my binge eating habit with as little stress as possible and make it as enjoyable as possible. I am here to tell you that, by using these same exact concepts, you can also break your binge eating habit.

We have already distinguished that, through quantum physics, your thoughts manifest into your physical world. I encourage you to be as creative as possible with your imagination, but the other piece to making manifestation work is putting your feelings into your thoughts and declarations, as if what you are trying to manifest already exists. We often forget the emotions that need to be part of what we are trying to manifest. Have you ever verbally declared that you would accomplish something, but didn't truly believe that it would happen or had doubt of it actually happening, and it ended up not happening? That's right nothing happened—that is exactly the result you manifested when your heart does not believe in your thoughts and in your declaration. Remember, we communicate with the quantum realm through both our thoughts and feelings. Both our thoughts and emotions have to work together to manifest the reality you want.

I am sure you have heard successful people say that in order to manifest and create the life you want, you must speak and declare the life you want on a daily base, engaging in daily affirmations. For example, if you want to be full of energy, claim and declare that you have an abundance of energy, right? Yes, of course, but you are only halfway there by speaking what you want into your life. I have learned the hard way. I practiced the concept of daily affirmations and verbally declaring what I wanted in my life for a very long time with no results. I even gave up for a while. I learned that simply declaring what

I wanted in my life would not work or didn't work as fast I would have hoped if I didn't truly believe my declarations with all my heart. Yes, verbally declaring what you want may help you move in the right direction because the Lord will attract to you what you have verbally declared. However, I have learned that verbally declaring your desires just isn't good enough. The secret to a successful manifestation is that you must imagine and speak the life you want to create into existence, and you must also truly feel it and believe in it your heart that you will and have already created the life you desire. When your heart and mind work together, you can truly create the life you desire.

Whatever you can imagine and want to manifest in your life, including breaking the habit of binge eating, believe it with all your heart that you got this, and that you are already living the life you dreamed of. So what if you have gone through many years of broken promises? Let this year be the year you keep your promises. We spend too much time and energy worrying about the "how" and "when" and not enough on what we want to manifest in our lives. The "how" will come—believe that God has the answer to your "how" and "when." Even if you spent twenty-four hours thinking about how things might play out, it would do you no good because a lot of things are out of our control. I would even go so far as to encourage you to give thanks as if you already have what you desire. This means giving thanks to finally setting yourself free of your binge eating habit, to your beautiful energetic body, to your healthy taste buds and cravings, and much more.

Recreating a Better Version of You

As you continue to create your desired physical reality by observing and influencing the energy around you, ultimately what you are doing is getting rid of your old thoughts and behaviors. You will also continue to create new thoughts and feelings that are in alignment with the person you want to become. This process is going to be an intentional process of creating the you that you have always wanted. You will have to continually and actively engage in your new thoughts and feelings. Once your new way of thinking and feeling becomes second nature, your new way of being follows naturally.

We are creatures of habit. Your body will want to tell you to revert to your old habits. In order to break your habit of binge eating, you need to understand how your brain and neurons work. For the most part, our subconscious mind directs our behaviors and belief systems, unless we are actively engaging with our conscious mind. Your mind should be in control of the way your body thinks and acts, not the other way around. But when you have been feeling and thinking a certain way for so many years, your body is conditioned to remember these same feelings and emotions, influencing your body to also react the same way, day in and day out. Your conscious mind will need to actively engage in self-reflection in order to redirect or refocus your old undesirable behaviors, which will lead you to create desired outcomes. These same feelings and emotions cause your brain to program the same circuits over and over again, eventually creating hardwired networks in the brain. Hardwired networks are essentially your subconscious mind.

These emotions furthermore create memorized chemicals that your body believes are the norm, and your body will want to resort back to them, making it hard to break your habit of binge eating. In other words, every time you give in to your short-lived temptations, your brain continues to tell the subconscious mind that this feels good and that these feelings and emotions are normal, ultimately creating the same memorized chemicals. But keep in mind that it only feels good and normal to the subconscious mind. Once the conscious mind kicks in, you then realize the damage you have done by binge eating once again, and the negative self-talk and feelings of frustration start to take over; adding to this never-ending binge eating cycle.

Think about this example; it will give you a better understanding of how and why our body wants to resort back to our old ways and habits. You had a great start to your day (and even ate a pretty healthy breakfast) that is, until you get to work. It's eleven o'clock—close to your lunchtime. Your mind starts to wander, and you think about what you want to eat for lunch. Automatically, your brain is drawn to the delicious burger and fries that you have been so used to eating, especially when work is constantly stressful (this is the start of your conditioned feelings and emotions influencing your actions and decisions). You start to imagine how it will taste and slowly melt in your mouth; you smell the delicious patty that is always cooked so perfectly. At some point, you can even hear the burger talking to you—it tells you this is what you have been craving all day, that you work so hard and you deserve it. If you don't fulfill your craving right now, your craving will continue to linger until you can finally indulge in your craving. It even tells you a little white lie about how the perfect time to eat it is now because as soon as you can eat it and get over this craving of yours, you can finally start your healthier lifestyle (this is where your conscious mind should have woken up and redirected your thoughts away from your favorite burger or stopped you from giving into your cravings, but instead, your conscious mind allows your subconscious and body to take over).

Even though your small, still voice wants you to resort to something healthier, like a salad, slowly but surely you will start to hear your subconscious mind talking to you (here you can see your conscious mind woke up just for two quick seconds and went back to sleep). Your subconscious mind and body will start to talk you out of a healthy lifestyle and your goals. You will start to tell yourself that it's been a stressful day and you deserve to cheat, just one more day (your conditioned emotions and feelings continue to take over and you continue to talk your way out of taking control of your binge eating habit today). You can always start tomorrow. Besides, today just wasn't a good day to start a healthier lifestyle. You will find any reason to cheat. It might be as simple as you prefer to start your healthier lifestyle on an even day versus an odd day. So, because it is January 19th and not 20th, it is definitely worth cheating one more day, and starting a healthier lifestyle on January 20th.

You continue to listen to your inner voice telling you to start today, right now. You successfully hit your lunch hour without binge eating. You even held off lunch until a little past noon. But your mind attempts one more time and continues to talk you out of your goals and continues to engage you in lusting over your favorite burger. Your mind digs deeper, coming up with more valid reasons as to why you deserve to give in to your favorite burger. Now you even start to beat yourself up. You tell yourself that you are stressed, not only is work stressful but your personal life adds to the stress. Your mom is never available, and you feel like you can never truly open up to her. You can't connect with your dad since their divorce years ago, and you are always feeling responsible for your two younger brothers who have had no one to depend on except you (this is your brain programming the same circuits, creating the same memorized chemicals and wanting to resort back to what feels normal). You continue to lust over your favorite burger and eventually let your reasoning and body win and give in. You indulge in your favorite burger and fries. By the time you can start to process what just happened, you realize that your goals once again went out the window. You already ate more than your body could handle; you are now regretting having given in to a temporary pleasure. You are frustrated and now beating yourself up, and find yourself in the middle of your never-ending binge eating cycle.

The goal is to refrain yourself from allowing your old, undesirable emotions and feelings influence your decisions or actions, which enables you to continue these cycles of binge eating. This involves making sure that you are engaging with your conscious mind as soon as you find yourself reverting back to your old feelings, thoughts, and habits. You want to engage your conscious mind in self-reflection and self-awareness. You want to make sure your conscious mind knows that these old actions, feelings, and thoughts are exactly what you should not and do not want to continue thinking about. By shifting your thoughts and through meditation, you want to engage your conscious mind to redirect your subconscious mind in activities, feelings, and thoughts that are aligned with the new you and your desired outcomes.

Once you engage in creating new thoughts and feelings, you can start to act upon these new thoughts, feelings, and actions; like committing to eating healthier or being able to control your binge eating. Acting upon these thoughts, feelings, and actions will also feel twice as easy, since you have already mentally rehearsed them through meditation. Your new decisions and actions will produce new feelings and emotions that will be aligned with the new and improved you; like feeling satisfied and energized after a nutritious meal. If you continue to engage in this new way of thinking and decision making, your brain will eventually start to re-program your circuits and this new way of thinking, feeling, and being will become second nature, and eventually the new you will begin to emerge naturally.

Using Meditation to Stop the Binge

In the next section, I will dive deeper into how you can create better outcomes when you are tempted to give in. You will learn to leverage and change your old, undesirable emotions and feelings through meditation to win over these binge eating battles.

There are three main ways in which I found quantum physics helpful in beating my own binge eating habit. Quantum physics can be used as a preventive measure to help you avoid binge eating, whenever you feel temptations and cravings creep up on you. With the second method, quantum physics can be used to help you get back on track, even if you happened to cheat. Remember, one cheat meal does not have to determine your future and does not have to deter you from all you have accomplished so far. The last method will allow you to play a proactive role in controlling your binge eating, you will be able influence your reality and will know exactly how to react when temptations and cravings arise. This method will teach you how to live as if you have already been living a successful binge-free life.

Let me introduce you to the concept of meditation. All of these methods can be accomplished through meditation. Meditation is a method of deep focus on a particular thought or activity. Meditation will allow you to lose yourself in thought and in time. Through meditation, you will be opening the door between the conscious and subconscious mind. The subconscious mind is where all of our habits and behaviors are stored, you want to access the subconscious mind in order to change your old, undesirable habits and behaviors to create the reality you desire.

Your purpose is to use meditation to focus on and rehearse the life you want: living binge-free. Of course, at some point, you will have to start taking action in your physical world to live the life you desire. But let me assure you that it starts in your mind. Not only will you start to see a physical manifestation, but starting with your mind will allow your journey to be easier and smoother. Remember that quantum physics is the endless possibility of energy that only comes to life when observed by you. By meditating, you will be able to think and feel your desires into reality.

Meditation to Avoid Binge Eating

It is important to understand you can improve a situation with meditation and mental rehearsal alone. It is also important to remember that to make the best use of meditation, you should be as proactive as possible, using meditation to help you avoid getting yourself into a continuous cycle of binge eating. Through the use of meditation, you will prepare yourself and know exactly how to react and respond when temptations and cravings come creeping up on you in your daily life. I am not guaranteeing that you will not make a mistake, but when you know how to react when temptations and cravings arise, you will be more prepared to turn them down and win each battle.

Meditation works because when you become so focused and concentrated on a particular thought or activity and truly put your whole heart into it, you will get to a place where your mind cannot distinguish if you are completing the task now, in the past, or in the future. Your mind goes to a place where it is no longer limited by time or space. Your mind and body think that you are performing the task as if you are presently engaged in the activity. The more you rehearse this particular thought or activity, the more you will sharpen your skills and knowledge, and eventually manifest it into life and understand exactly what you need to do to complete the task.

There have been multiple studies to show that mentally rehearsing and mentally practicing a specific task improves performance and improves progress. A study conducted on patients with chronic strokes showed that the group who completed mental practice in addition to their therapy session exhibited greater reductions in their impairments, compared to the patients who only completed therapy sessions without engaging in mental practice. Another recent study revealed that mental practice before performing surgery improved a surgeon's technical ability and enhanced their performance.

The following will give you an example of how your mind can take you to a place where you are not limited by time or space. Let's take, for example, your relationship with your mom. You have been bitter at your mom for so long. After your parents' divorce, when you were ten years old, your mom has neglected you and your brothers, and your feelings. Even more recently, she had the nerve to embarrass you by talking horribly about you in front of your whole family and her close friends. You've been constantly thinking about this incident since it happened almost a month ago. Every time you think about it, you seem to get just as mad and frustrated as if it just happened yesterday. You start to clench your jaw, you can feel a headache coming on, your heart starts racing, and you get irritated at anything and everything around you. Your mind gets so fired up by your past emotions and event that it forgets that you are actually not engaged in the actual event at the moment; you are no longer limited by space or time. Similarly, you can engage yourself in meditation with the same amount of concentration and emotion. This concentrated meditation will take you to a place where you are no longer limited by space or time, and your brain will not be able to distinguish whether or not you are actually physically engaged in the activity.

Now, let's take what you just learned about engaging in mental rehearsal and meditation and turn it into something positive. You can use mental rehearsal and meditation to help you get out of the rut of binge eating. Remember our previous example of how our body wants to resort back to binge eating? When eleven o'clock hits, even on your most stressful day, you want to use what you have just learned about engaging in concentrated meditation and reprogramming your brain's hardwired networks to control binge eating. Instead of lustfully thinking about your favorite burger and fries, you want to meditate and lust over those fresh strawberries that you brought from home and that homemade honey garlic chicken thigh you made with love and gratitude. Of course, it might be only natural for your brain to revert back to your favorite burger. After all, your body and its memorized chemicals want you to resort back to that short-lived pleasure it is used to. You have no control when your brain reverts back to your favorite burger, however, you do have control over how long you allow your brain to continue to lust over your favorite burger. Your goal is to engage your conscious mind to redirect your thoughts back to those yummy vitamin-filled strawberries and honey garlic chicken as soon as possible. This is when your brain wants to start talking you out of your goals, and you will also want to take a few moments to call upon the Lord. Ask the Lord to renew your mind to what is good and nutritious for you. Calling on the Lord doesn't have to be anything that should take up extra time. All you do is, as soon as you start hearing your mind start to justify why you should give up your healthy lifestyle, you meditate and repeat God's truth. It goes something like this:

> *Lord please renew my mind to all that is good and nutritious for me. Please help me to think and act accordingly so that I can continue to build a healthy and strong temple for myself and a temple for the Holy Spirit to reside in. Amen!*

Remember how it was so natural and easy for you to use all your senses when reminiscing about how your favorite burger would taste in your mouth and how you could smell that perfectly cooked patty miles away? When meditating, you also need to retrain your brain to think in the same way, using all five of your senses. All five senses should be used to reminisce about your delicious strawberries and homemade honey garlic chicken. Take some time to imagine how those fresh strawberries and that honey garlic chicken would taste and slowly melt in your mouth, how they would smell, and how such a nutritious meal is calling your name, waiting to nourish your body.

In addition to meditation, remember all the reasonings and pep-talks you gave yourself justifying why you should give in and cheat as soon as you are hungry, and your cravings start calling you? That's exactly what you need to put into practice with a positive twist to it so that you can create an environment supportive of your healthier and binge-free lifestyle. Your pep-talk and reasoning should go something like this:

> *Even though it's been a stressful morning, I am making the decision to love myself and fuel my body with nutritious*

food. I deserve a body that is strong, beautiful, and properly operating. I am so glad today is the perfect day to start my new healthy, healing lifestyle. I am healthy. I am full of energy and life. I am worthy. I am happy and confident in my progress so far. I am in control of my eating habits and my emotions. Nothing is impossible for me. I have a loving and supportive family that is blessed beyond measures.

Can you see just how much more powerful this last pep-talk (versus beating yourself up) will be in helping you to free yourself from binge eating? I encourage you to do this daily, especially when temptations and cravings arise. It becomes easier with practice, especially when you truly believe it with all your heart that nutritious food is just as good, delicious, and fulfilling as your favorite burger.

I had a client named Liz who found her husband using this same positive pep-talk method I taught her. Liz's husband became her accountability partner. Liz was a very verbal and outgoing person. She started using this positive pep-talk method out loud every time she felt cravings and temptations creeping up on her. Two months into using this method, on a Saturday evening, without thinking, she was trying to justify out loud why she deserved to cave into all her cravings tonight. She was surprised when her husband started giving her the positive pep-talk. He told her it was fine to have one or two slices of pizza, but would be unwise to completely give in and eat everything (which she used to do). He continued to tell her that she had come too far to completely give in. He told her she was beautiful, and continues to become even more beautiful, both inside and out (this was, according to Liz, obviously because of the new found energy she started having). He continued to tell her that she deserved to feel beautiful, powerful, and so much more.

Using Quantum Physics After a Cheat Meal

Remember, this is going to be a lifestyle change that you are creating for yourself. Let's face it, you are not perfect. No one is. The truth is, you are going to make mistakes throughout your journey. This means that along the way, you may find yourself periodically giving in and having yourself a cheat meal. I understand that you have been making broken promises to yourself, and at this point, you are totally fed up. But beating yourself up and feeling guilty isn't going to fix anything and it sure isn't going to create the life you want. Remember, what you observe, you create. After giving into a cheat meal, if you observe that you are worthless and that you will never overcome binge eating, that is exactly what you will be creating for your future.

Your meditation after a cheat meal should be as soon as you can squeeze in a few minutes to meditate. Meditating will help you clear your mind and even release the disappointment you are probably feeling in yourself. Your meditation should be focused on forgiving yourself, moving on without guilt, and rehearsing the cheat meal that just happen and how you will approach those cravings and temptations differently next time. Even if you are not able to squeeze in some time to meditate, you must be aware of the words you are speaking to yourself.

Your self-talk after a cheat meal is probably negative; you need to keep those thoughts and self-talks positive. I will teach you how remaining positive looks like.

I want you to clearly understand that I believe it is completely fine to feel your emotions after you have indulged in an unhealthy meal. It is only natural to be disappointed with yourself after ruining your awesome progress so far. Take a minute or two to feel your emotions, even cry it out if you have to. But as soon as your two minutes are up, you need to get right back on track, so that you can continue creating the life you want. You need to simply feel your emotions, but avoid at all costs mentally and verbally beating yourself up. Remember, beating yourself up will create the life you have been wanting to get away from.

Your self-talk should go a little like this, even after feeling horrible about giving in and indulging in your favorite junk food:

Geez, I can't believe I ruined my progress. I am so mad at myself. I can't continue to do this every time I am with friends and family. Aahhh (swear a little, if you have to)!

At this point, you will naturally want to resort to beating yourself up and talking down to yourself. Remember, negative self-talk will create a cycle of the negative emotions you are used to feeling. You will probably want to tell yourself that you are worthless, ugly, and fat, and will never amount to anything.

But instead of beating yourself up, you need to take a deep breath and tell yourself:

Okay. You know what? I got this. I am in control of what I put in my body. I have come so far and made so much progress. Thank you, Lord. I am wonderfully and beautifully made. I am energized. I am totally worth this and my mistake does not determine my future.

The first time you talk to yourself positively after a cheat meal, it may feel a bit weird because you are used to beating yourself up. But keep it positive and keep meditating on those positive thoughts until you feel them and truly believe in them. Smile a little—this will definitely help brighten your mood and change your brain's memorized chemicals in the right direction to help keep you pushing forward.

Jessica came to me because no matter what she did, she found herself constantly giving in and continuing her binge eating cycles. She informed me that even after she started implementing positive self-talk and meditation, starting a healthy lifestyle and committing to it was almost impossible. I had to ask her if she truly believed in her meditation and positive self-talk with all her heart. I had to remind her that even if she promised herself that she would stop cheating, if she did not truly believe she could, manifesting the reality she wanted may be impossible. As she slowly learned how to put her heart and feelings into truly believing she would stop cheating and finally start living a life filled with good health and energy, her cheat meals became few and far between.

Using Quantum Physics Daily to Produce Results

If you are anything like me, you like a fast-paced life and might find meditation a bit boring, intimidating, or even just nearly impossible to do. It's going to take practice and my hope is that eventually you will learn to love it, like I did. The more I started to manifest things into my physical reality, the more I looked forward to meditating. It's actually how I spend a lot of my "me" time now. Meditation always seems to have a way of calming me down and renewing my mind and soul.

The goal is to meditate daily in order to help you use the energy around you to create the life you want—to create a life that will support you in taking control of your binge eating habits with less hassle and frustration. Creating what you desire means focusing your meditation on a life as if you are already eating when you want and what you want without any feelings of guilt, frustration, or discouragement because it is healthy, delicious food.

It took me a while to know exactly what I should focus my meditation on to get the results I wanted in becoming binge-free. I will show you exactly what you need to meditate on in order to manifest your desired results. Especially when starting out, you should focus your meditation on one desired result at a time. For example, you may really want to manifest both being free of binge eating and a better relationship with your parents, but start off slowly, first focusing on being in control of binge eating. It's a lifelong process, but once you get the hang of it, you will be able to manifest other things into reality. I encourage you to start with my guidelines until you start to get the hang of it. Because you are a unique individual with unique goals and desires, you will eventually want to take your imagination above and beyond what I give you. Only you know what you want and what is best for you.

You can meditate either in the morning right after you wake up, when your mind is still fresh, or right before bedtime when you are winding down for the night. I highly recommend you incorporate this as part of your morning routine. When you start meditating, I would suggest starting with meditating for ten to fifteen minutes; this will help build your endurance and focus during meditation. You can always meditate longer once you feel comfortable enough.

For a long time, I was meditating at night simply because I am not a morning person. Once I started a morning routine, I started to incorporate meditation in the morning. I found that my morning routine that includes meditation and prayer sets my mood and emotion for the day. Trust me, coming from a person who despises early mornings, creating a morning routine for yourself is definitely worth it.

Your first few minutes should be spent settling into your meditation, trying to reach what I call your zone of genesis. To find your zone of genesis, you want to find a place that is comfortable enough to focus, but not too comfortable that you will fall asleep. It would be best if you sat cross-legged with your body, back, and head as straight as possible. Get comfortable. Set a timer for ten to fifteen minutes. Put on some relaxing instrumental music that will help get you focused. Music can definitely vary from person to person or even day to day. Tune in to how you are feeling that day. It is important to choose music with no lyrics because what may happen is that your mind may start to focus on the lyrics and distract you from your purpose for meditation. Start your meditation by deeply breathing in and out. Focus on your breath. As you focus on your breath, you will want to either focus on an image or activity. You will know you have gotten to your zone of genesis when you have lost yourself deep into thought and meditation with no awareness of yourself or time. You will simply be present in your meditation; at this point, your mind should not be able to distinguish whether or not you are actually completing the activity.

You can choose to either focus your meditation on an image or an activity. Focusing my meditation on an image many times means meditating on how much leaner my body is looking as I look at myself in my bedroom mirror or how much more energy I have while I am in my Zumba class. As you begin your meditation journey, your focused activity should be meditating on a day in your life, living as if you have already broken free from binge eating. If you cannot rehearse or meditate your whole day within the ten to fifteen minutes window, don't worry. Remember, do not waste your energy worrying about unnecessary details, like the "how" and "when."

You will start with envisioning yourself waking up. You will also envision what you are eating throughout the day. You will go through your work day and any temptations that come along, meditating on how you will react to your temptations and cravings. Keep in mind that you do not want to be the same you that you have always been—giving in to your temptations and cravings. You want to create a new being. This means that you will want to react in a way that is different from the way you have always reacted. Imagine yourself being in control and successfully conquering your temptations.

When meditating, remember to use your five senses—smell your fresh cooked food and feel your energized body. Meditation is meant for you to be as creative as you can be. Meditation may go a little like this:

I see myself waking up and getting ready for the day on a positive note. My body feels amazing. I take a peek in the mirror and my toned, flexible body is smiling back at me, ready to take on the day. I brush my teeth, wash my face, and take a moment to smile at myself in the mirror, delighted at my progress so far. I walk into my office where I start my daily routine. After my daily routine, I'm on my way to the kitchen and making myself my morning green tea. I peek into the fridge and see a whole lot of food options, both good and bad because my husband has not completely jumped on the healthy lifestyle with me. I move past the bacon, and reach for an apple and strawberries. I reach for some eggs and close my fridge. I start to smell my organic eggs frying in the background. I am feeling so excited because as I look at my watch, I even made enough time this morning to make my own homemade lunch. I sit down to have a little prayer time, finish my breakfast and pop some chicken breast into the oven for lunch before I go and get ready for my work day. Once I return to the kitchen, my chicken smells amazing and looks quite juicy. As I am preparing my salad for lunch, I can smell its freshness. I even take some time to imagine how delicious this salad will be once lunchtime comes. I tell myself I cannot wait to fuel my body with such goodness. I continue to see myself at work and taking on my morning. Eleven o'clock hits, my mind automatically thinks about my favorite burger, but I refocus my thoughts on the salad and chicken breast I have already made. I image how delicious and fresh my salad is going to taste, and, more importantly, how energized I will feel after lunch. Four o'clock hits, I mentally start planning for a healthy dinner. I run through what I had in my fridge this morning, and determine if I might have to run to the grocery store to get something. By dinner time, my husband and I are eating my deliciously cooked meal together, discussing our day, and even planning for a date night. When eight p.m. rolls around, this is the time I usually get my late-night sweet tooth cravings. I imagine myself going to the freezer to look for my usual go-to ice cream that I love so much. I pause, I think about how far I have come, I close the freezer door and decided to put on some music to pump me up so that I can go to the gym, instead of eating that ice cream, even if going to the gym just means going to sit in the sauna far from my temptation. My upbeat music keeps me going in the sauna. I come back from the gym, my cravings have disappeared, and now I am ready to relax for the night.

See how simple that was? Remember, you got this! Commit to meditating daily, and it will get easier.

Quantum Physics Alignment with God

When I started learning about quantum physics, I noticed some similarities and alignments quantum physics had with the word of God. This was important to me because in my process of seeking healing and recovery from binge eating, I also knew that above all else is ultimately God's truth, His will, and His purpose for me. I also knew that willpower alone was not going to work. I have tried using my willpower for so many years without much success. When I came upon quantum physics and found its alignment with God's words, I knew this was the tool God wanted me to use to help me conquer my binge eating habit. Below are the alignments I noticed. These alignments not only remind me to continue to immerse myself in God's words, but also keeps me engaged in meditation so that I can manifest in my life all things that are prosperous and wonderful, including my health.

> *"Do not conform to the pattern of this world,*
> *but be transformed by the renewing of your mind."*
> **– Romans 12:2**

The process of using quantum physics is a process of renewing your mind, creating a new being and reality for yourself. Similarly, God wants us to continually renew our minds and let go of the worldly desires and addictions, such as food, so that we can live out the purpose He has for us. Renewal of the mind will also allow us to enjoy and love our temple the Lord has fearfully and wonderfully made. We have been made perfectly in God's creation and image; therefore we should not doubt His creation, but continue to reserve and optimize this temple He has given to us. God wants us to keep our temples as healthy and functional as possible so that the Holy Spirit can have a peaceful place to call home.

> *"Above all else, guard your heart,*
> *for everything you do flows from it."*
> **– Proverbs 4:23**

We have previously discussed how much more you can manifest the life you want when you truly believe in your declarations and thoughts with all our heart. This aligns with what the Lord tells us as He wants us to guard our hearts above all else. He wants us to know that our thoughts and our declarations have the power to affect us. Therefore, you must be careful about what you speak and think. This means no more beating yourself up over your mistakes, and no more speaking or thinking about what you do not want to manifest in your life. The Lord only wants you to think about things that are good and pure.

> *"This is the message we have heard from Him and declare*
> *to you: God is light; in Him there is no darkness at all."*
> **– 1 John 1:5**

Quantum physics teaches us that we cannot think a certain way and feel another and expect change to happen. The mind and the heart must be one. This means that even if you declare that you will not give into temptations at your next potluck, but still have doubt, your desired outcomes will not manifest. You must truly believe it and feel it—no doubt or second-guessing. With all the meditation you have completed, you should have no problem knowing how you plan to tackle each temptation. Similarly, God states that where there is light, there is no darkness. You simply cannot succeed with positive thoughts, but a doubtful heart; both of them cannot exist at the same time. Allow God to be your light so that your dark days can be behind you. Ask Him to guide you in each situation and each temptation that comes your way. Ask Him to show you how to be positive. Where there is God and light, temptations become so much easier to tackle.

> *"Therefore I tell you, whatever you ask for in prayer, believe that you have received it, and it will be yours."*
> **– Mark 11:24**

You meditate so you can create your physical reality by observing the energy around you. During meditation, you are to focus as if you already have exactly what you want or what you have prayed for. You are to speak and think with gratitude as if you already have it. Let's face it, we are not grateful for something we have not received. The Lord wants you to know that you have already received it. He says that when you ask, believe you have already received it. Live as if you have already received it. The battle has already been won. Know that whatever you ask for, it shall be given to you according to His will. Whatever you ask for may not come in the form you hope for, nor will it come when you want it to come, but be confident because it is already yours. When I want something from the Lord, I spend less time asking for it and more time thanking Him for it. I will go to the Lord with my problem and put in my request once or twice (just to make sure He hears my request) but after that, I thank Him for already giving it to me. A good example is that I no longer go to the Lord to ask for healing, I simply state "Thank you Lord through your stripes I am healed!"

> *"Do not be anxious about anything, but in every situation, by prayer and petition, with thanksgiving, present your requests to God. And the peace of God, which transcends all understanding, will guard your hearts and your minds in Christ Jesus."*
> **– Philippians 4:6—4:7**

As humans, we are so used to wanting to be in control all the time. You spend so much time worrying about the "how" and "when" that you forget to continue using that energy towards creating the life you want. Quantum physics and God teach us that we need to trust the Lord and leave the "how" and "when" up to Him. God will not only give you what you ask for, but He will give you above and beyond all you can ever imagine or ask for. When you finally give up trying to control and understand the "how" and "when," you receive a peace from God that confirms no matter how long it takes, it will be done.

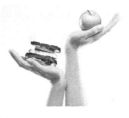

Chapter 4

Understanding God's Promises for Me

In the world we live in, where health crises seem to be on the rise and gun violence and other horrific violence continue to threaten our world, we now need God more than ever. It is more important than ever to actively reach out to God and invite Him into your journey to better health so that you can finally be in control of your binge eating.

It is important that you learn to tune into what He is saying to you and tune into His guidance and promises that He wants you to receive. Perhaps sometimes, when it seems like you don't hear Him, it is because you haven't been tuning into His words, and perhaps other times you don't hear Him because He is testing your faith and obedience. The Lord wants you to stay engaged in his words and His truth. He wants you to know that He is a God of healing, not just of the past, but of today. He wants you to trust that He will guide you through the storm ahead and to show you that even in deep waters, He will be there to lift you up.

My Identity in Christ

During my endless cycles of binge eating, I found myself digging deeper into a state a depression, as I often engaged in a cycle of verbally and mentally beating myself up with negative self-talk. These talks led to more frustration, confusion, and depression. I would continue to tell myself day-in and day-out that I was ugly and fat; I was useless; how could I do this to myself again; I was never going to follow through; how stupid I was and how out of control I was. I told myself these things, not realizing how much these words and thoughts affected my mind, body, and life.

I found myself at a breaking point and was fed up with my negative self-talk. At this point, I was also in the middle of getting to know God. I was just recently re-introduced to having God in my life, but I found myself drawing closer to Him because I knew I couldn't do this by myself. I needed the Lord to help me with my binge eating habits, a healthier lifestyle, and with healing.

At my breaking point, I started to discover my true identity in the Lord. Through my identity that came from the Lord, I discovered what He truly thought of me and how He saw me. The more I focused on my identity that was rooted in

Him, the less I focused on my own identity of myself and the identity other people gave me. This helped reduce my negative self-talk. Every time I would resort to negative self-talk, I had to continually remind myself of God's truth and my identity I found in Him in order to realize that I am worth it, and that I can be in control of my binge eating.

In the Lord, I found these truths that helped me identify who I was to the Lord. I hope that you will learn these truths also apply to you, and encourage you to discover your own identity in the Lord.

- I am a daughter of God and deserve all things that are wonderfully made. All things will work together for my good.
- If God heals my brothers and sisters, He will heal me, too. I deserve it just as much as anyone else because He loves me just as much as He loves them.
- I am beautiful. I am fearfully and wonderfully made. He took his time to craft me exactly how He wanted me to be. I am not perfect, but God has made me exactly as I should be. In Him is my new creation and life.
- God is forgiving. Even if I continue to make mistakes, God will continue to love me and forgive me. If God can forgive me, I should also forgive myself.
- Only God can judge me and define me. I will be respectful of other people's opinion of me, but I will not allow anyone to define me, nor will I let any worldly attributes define me.

- My body is my temple. The Holy Spirit dwells in it, I must glorify God in how I treat this temple that He has given me.
- I can do all things through God because He will give me the strength, peace, and grace I need to overcome my binge eating habits.

Don't Throw Yourself a Self-Pity Party!

It is extremely important for you to take some time to take care of yourself. I would even encourage you to make it a habit of setting aside time to take care of yourself daily. Do this by creating a morning or evening routine; something you can truly commit to. We can both agree that life gets busy, and sometimes it seems impossible to squeeze in time for yourself, but the truth is we all are given twenty-four hours in a day. Even if it means waking up a little bit earlier or staying up a little bit later, it will be totally worth it. I recommend spending some time taking care of yourself to rejuvenate so that you can be your best version of yourself for both you and your loved ones. This will also ensure you go through life full of energy, and free yourself from simply going through the motions in life. You don't want to wait until physical symptoms start to show up before taking care of yourself; most of the time, that means that you have already outdone yourself.

However, it is not okay to take time in your daily life to throw yourself a self-pity party. I learned that being pitiful and powerful takes the same amount of energy, so I could either choose to be pitiful or powerful. I chose powerful. I hope you will, too.

This means stop living in the past! Stop feeling sorry for yourself, and stop regretting experiences and events that happened in the past. It happened. Move on. There is nothing you can do to change it. What you can do is take that time to focus on changing your future and taking care of yourself.

As we previously discussed, it helps when you are able to find your identity in the Lord. This will help you stop any self-pity party you decide to throw for yourself, including negative talk, negative thoughts, and negative actions, like binge eating. Talk to yourself as if you believe you are a daughter of God, as if He is talking to you. You are His daughter and He wants you to be successful. Anytime you find yourself talking negatively or thinking negatively, you need to ask the Lord to help you think of only positive thoughts. The Lord wants you to set our minds on "... whatever is true, whatever is noble, whatever is right, whatever is pure, whatever is lovely, whatever is admirable..." (Philippians 4:8, New International Version) and you should do just that.

Early on in my journey, I found myself throwing self-pity parties quite often because I did not understand God's promises for me. The more I understood His promises and actually had faith that His promises would come to pass, the less frustrated I felt and the fewer self-pity parties I engaged in. Some of the promises the Lord has taught me that helped reduced my self-pity parties are:

- I need to obey His command and do my part to the best of my abilities, but I do not need to try to be in control of everything. I need to be still and wait patiently and allow the Lord to do His part also. This means that, for me, I should do my best to feed my body all the good, nutritious food God has created. Everything else is in God's hands and He will do His part in healing me. I need to trust that He will take care of it.

- If I lack wisdom, I shall ask. The Lord will give me wisdom generously, regardless of any of my past sins. When I started my journey, I lacked so much wisdom and resources, but all I had to do was ask, and it was given to me. Most of the time, His wisdom did not come exactly the way I was hoping for or at the exact time I was hoping for, but it took a lot of learning and understanding that I need to trust that He knows best and will give me the wisdom I need when I need it. I also learned that God knows exactly what I need and will provide for me even before I can ask for it.

- "I called to the Lord, who is worthy of praise, and I have been saved from my enemies." (Psalm 18: 3, New International Version) This doesn't mean that there will be no temptations, nor does this mean that I will not be faced with challenges. It does mean that when I call on the Lord and understand that He is bigger and stronger than any temptations or problems I face, I shall win any and all battles and struggles that come my way.

- I am my own worst critic. Even when no one is judging me or comparing themselves to me, I am always comparing myself to others. I found myself many times a bit jealous as to why that person was able to control their eating habit, why he or she got what I have always wanted for myself, and I even started to wonder if God was choosing favorites or honoring other people's prayers and not mines. I had to learn in order to truly trust God and His timing, I must be happy exactly where I am. I had to learn to be happy for others because God will only give me as much as I can handle. This was the only way I was truly ever going to be happy and be at peace with myself, my journey, and what I was already so blessed with.

Are You Spiritually Starving?

Have you ever been in a situation where you just ate a full meal, but feel like you were still hungry or something was still missing from the meal you just had? This happened quite often when I first started my journey. Sometimes I would go about scavenging through my fridge to see what else I could possibly try to eat, hoping not to overstuff myself. I slowly learned, through experiences similar to this one where no matter how much I ate I still felt empty, that I might be spiritually starving and not actually physically hungry. I have learned that spiritual hunger comes along with mood swings and emotional instability. Things just seem out of balance and very chaotic, even if I was doing everything right in life. I often felt confused, irritable, and could not get myself to focus. I had to slowly learn through my relationship with God that no food, no matter how much I ate, could ever satisfy my soul.

If you want to stay physically healthy, most of us have to intentionally stay active and eat well. Similarly, if you want to be spiritually well, you must also intentionally stay active in His words and feed your soul with His words. Nowadays, when I start to feel emotionally imbalanced, I turn to the Lord's words. You can spiritually feed your soul anywhere and anytime. In most places that you can eat, you can also feed your spiritual soul. You can even spiritually feed your soul right at work as often as you need, especially on a stressful day. All you have to do is ask the Lord to fill you with his words, allow this hunger to go away, get yourself a cup of water or tea, and pull out your bible, devotional app, or search for his words on the internet. It should take no more than a few minutes. After you are done feeding on his words, you should feel at peace and so much calmer. Many times, within the few minutes that you are feeding on his words, your hunger pain seems to magically disappear.

I encourage you to practice feeding on God's words to support you in breaking your binge eating habit. As you know, feeling stressed and emotionally unstable will give you all the reasons that sound like great reasons to give in to temptations. Feeding on God's words will allow you to become more emotionally centered, allowing you to make better decisions that are not based on how you are currently feeling at the moment. God's words will not leave you scavenging through the fridge to fill your starving soul.

Experiencing Spiritual Maturity

Once you find yourself grounded in God's truth and have enough faith to believe His promises for you, you will start to find yourself experiencing spiritual maturity. This does not mean that you have graduated from God and that you will no longer need to rely on God or feed on His words daily. This simply means that you can use your growth and spiritual maturity to deepen your relationship with the Lord, and use it so you can continue to live a binge-free life and experience deeper healing.

What exactly is spiritual maturity and how do you know when you have reached it, you ask? Besides aligning yourself with God's words and obeying His command, spiritual maturity is similar to human maturity. When we hit our teen years, we all felt as if our parents and the world were against us. When we reach a level of maturity, we realize that everything our parents did for us and said to us was to protect and guide us. Similarly, before the Lord and before understanding what His promises are to you, you probably felt that your world was crashing down on you, everybody was always against you, you always had to put your guard up, and believed people were out to hurt you. But once you understand the Lord's truth and receive His grace, all those negative feelings and perceptions of the world turn positive. What was once fear turns into peace; anger turns into happiness; sorrow turns into joy; and the biggest one for me was when hate turned into love.

At one point, I was so bitter with the people in my life. They just seem to continue to hurt me. It caused me a lot of stress and it was eating away at me mentally and emotionally. It took a long time for me to learn that hurt people hurt others to feel better. Maybe they were hurting themselves and did not know how to handle their hurt. I also learned that I had to separate their sins from the person they were because God does the same for me. I was surprised by the grace and strength the Lord gave me to forgive the people in my life that have hurt me. One day, I found myself praying for those who had hurt me and caused me so much bitterness to be healed. It definitely wasn't that I hated them one day, and came to love them overnight, but wishing them well was a huge step in the right direction.

Being able to reach spiritual maturity and letting go of my bitterness and hurt also allowed me to better tackle my binge eating habit. When I was an emotional mess from all the hurt, I found so many justifications and reasons to binge eat. My emotions definitely controlled what I ate that day. When I was stressed or emotional, I found myself giving into binge eating much more easily. If I was emotionally stable, I was less likely to give in that day, and I ate healthier. Emotional stability definitely allowed me to have more control over what I ate.

It is critical to understand that spiritual maturity comes with time. It took me at least five years to finally be able to pray for those who hurt me. The more you feed on the Lord's words, align yourself with His words, and obey His commands, the more growth you will see in yourself. However, spiritual maturity doesn't just come when you choose for it to come, nor does it come overnight or in one sitting. It's a process, but I assure you that once you experience spiritual maturity. there is no way to miss it.

Lord, What Is Holding Me Back?

In the midst of trying to take control of my binge eating habit, I still found myself cheating and giving in some days and eating just horribly. I am that type of person, where once I give in, I want to eat everything in sight. Before giving in, I often found myself trying to justify why I should give in. I started to realize my reasons and justification for cheating were more than just giving into my actual craving. Most of my justifications were based on negative beliefs I had about food. Beliefs that actually held me back from finally reaching my goal of freeing myself from these binge eating cycles.

In frustration, I went to God and I prayed this simple prayer to the Lord asking Him for guidance.

> *Dear Lord,*
>
> *Please help me understand and reveal to me anything that is holding me back from successfully breaking my binge eating habit. Please reveal to me any beliefs I have about food that is holding me back. Please guide me and reveal to me your truth.*
>
> *In Jesus' name.*
>
> *Amen!*

My hope is that you will also use this prayer to discover what beliefs you have about food that have been holding you back from successfully breaking your binge eating habit. This may be a process that takes more than one sitting to completely understand the negative beliefs you have about food that has been holding you back. Keep in mind, God only gives you as much as you can handle.

I encourage you to set some time to pray this prayer and listen to that small, still voice—that is the Holy Spirit communicating with you. I would encourage you to journal all that you hear from the Lord. My experience is that when the Lord speaks to me, He makes sure I know it is Him who is speaking because He makes sure the details and knowledge

He gives me are above and beyond my own knowledge and understanding. I love writing down what the Lord reveals to me because at a later time when I need some guidance or advice, I can always go back and meditate on His wisdom and His promises for me.

Through that one simple, but desperate prayer, below are the truths the Lord revealed to me in order for me to gain a new perspective on my beliefs about food. Every time I caught myself justifying why I should give in to binge eating, I would repeat these truths that were revealed to me. These truths helped me to stop my habit of justifying why I should give in to binge eating. I hope these truths will help you gain a new perspective about food and will encourage you to reach out to the Lord to discover your own negative beliefs you have about food.

- God shall provide all my needs, including food. Food will not run out—there will always be plenty of food. Growing up with nine siblings, I learned that if I did not eat fast enough, I was likely not to get my second serving of food. This led me to believe as a young child that there may not be enough food, or if I didn't indulge in whatever I was craving or whatever food was available, I would not get the chance to eat it later. The Lord has taught me that there will always be enough food, and food will always be available. You will get a second serving if you feel you need it. He also taught me that, even if I do not get to eat that one piece of cake I was craving and was also available today, I can eat it at a later time and it will still be available. I might have to cook it myself, but it will always be available. I can indulge in my craving at a later time, after I meet my goals (whether that is being in control of my eating, losing two more pounds, or feeling more energized). I now understand that it feels better and is more meaningful when I indulge in my craving as more of a celebration of my accomplishments, instead of simply giving in.

- God will give me choices, including food choices, but not everything is a good choice for me. Are the foods I am choosing to put in my body glorifying God? Once I understood this, any time I put something in my mouth, I have learned to ask myself whether this food would both glorify God and also preserve and nurture the temple He has given me.

- Embrace hunger. Our bodies were designed not only to thrive in fullness, but also in hunger. The more I embraced hunger, the better I felt. I always come out of embracing hunger, when extending my fasting hours, more energized, focused, and refreshed. This truly gave me a glimpse into why Jesus fasted when He was seeking a break-through.

- Invite God to dine with me. God has a table waiting for me. He is my Father and desires to dine with me. He wants to have a conversation with me and wants to bless this temple of mine. I don't know about you, but I am a fast eater. I have found that when I do ask the Lord to dine with me, I tend to eat slower and actually

take time to enjoy my food. I am also less distracted by
the busyness of life when I dine with the Lord.

The negative beliefs each one of us have about food that
the Lord reveals never cease to amaze me. Every time I work
with a client through this activity, each client has such unique
and different beliefs about food that have been holding them
back. I had a client named Jamie. Jamie had always been a
heavier-set gal. She expressed to me that, as young as she could
remember, her mother has always reminded her not to eat too
much or she would get fat. She eventually learned not to eat a
lot in front of people, including her husband, but would binge
eat alone. She constantly looked forward to the time she could
be alone and eat her heart out. In one of our session together,
the Lord taught her that it was okay to eat until she was
satisfied in front of people. This will avoid having her starve
all day and finally binge eat once she was alone. She learned
that eating when she was hungry, even if it meant eating with
people around, would help her better manage her binge eating
habit. She should not have to feel that the only time she could
truly be fulfilled by food was when she was by herself in one of
her binge eating sessions.

A Five-Step Plan to Break Free of Binge Eating

In my short years of knowing the Lord and battling my own
binge eating habit, I have come to discover steps that I know I
can turn to in order to get back on track with creating a healthier
lifestyle. I used these steps often when I felt stuck, frustrated, or
in another cycle of horrible eating. I am not perfect and found

myself in the cycle of giving in too many times as I battled this addiction, but as soon as I could spend time with the Lord going through these steps, I got back on track. I have used this process both in this same exact order and other times out of order; as a quick go-to to get myself back on track. My suggestion is that, because you are just starting out, you should complete one step each day over a period of five days, in the exact order I have presented here, until you are comfortable enough with switching these steps around.

Day 1: Going to the Lord

The Lord loves it when you humble yourself before Him. This lets Him know that you need Him, and you are dependent on Him. When I go to the Lord humbly, I go to Him on my knees in prayer. I let Him know of my binge eating habit that I just can't seem to fight by myself. I confess to Him my sin of treating this temple He has given me horribly. I apologize for allowing food to control me and allowing food to become my idol, instead of focusing on the Lord and turning to Him. Let it be known that you are going to Him for help because you cannot do this alone.

Day 2: Releasing Strongholds

Most of the time, when we can't get over a habit or addiction, it is because we have a spiritual stronghold locking us down. A spiritual stronghold is a lie that the devil has told you, which usually derives from a past hurt or past negative experience you have had. You believe in these lies so much, it is ingrained in you, and it is impossible to distance yourself from it without

God's grace. Strongholds may reflect your beliefs about yourself or about the Lord. Strongholds will cause you to think in ways which will block you from God and His truth.

Go to the Lord today and ask Him to release you from all your strongholds that have been holding you down. If you are aware of some of your strongholds, specifically ask Him to release those strongholds. However, it is impossible for you to know all of your strongholds that are holding you down, but God is aware of all of them. Ask Him to release any other strongholds that you are not aware of that are holding you back from taking control of binge eating.

Day 3: Wisdom and Guidance

Ask the Lord today for wisdom and guidance so that you can break free from your binge eating cycles. Ask Him to renew your mind to all that is good and pure. Ask to be led by the Holy Spirit on this journey. This is also a great time to ask Him to help you change your taste buds to all that is healthy; so that you can learn to love and crave healthier foods. Go ahead and ask Him to help you distinguish your spiritual hunger from your physical hunger. You can also ask Him to give you resources or connections that will support you in breaking your binge eating habit.

Day 4: Guide My Emotions

You have learned you continually repeat these binge eating cycles because you allow your emotions to make rash decisions for you. Today is the day you are going to ask the Lord to guide your emotions.

Ask Him to give you peace and grace so that you do not make rash decisions and end up in the midst of the same binge eating cycles. Ask Him to guide your feelings and emotions. There are going to be times when you do not seem to hear or feel God's presence, ask Him to teach you to go beyond your emotions and feelings, so that you can continue to obey His commands and guidance. Even when you are emotional and feeling frustrated, fearful, and uncertain, ask the Lord to remind you to never confirm these negative emotions with your mouth but use your mouth to only agree with God's truth and His promises for you.

Day 5: Only God Can Set You Free

On this very last day, go to the Lord and ask Him to give you words to live by and to meditate on so you can get rid of this addiction once and for all. Continue to meditate on His words, especially when you feel the devil is attacking you. Be prepared to experience more spiritual warfare because the devil will attack harder when he knows that you are on your way to winning this battle. Let God know you believe He is the only one who can set you free. Remind yourself He is the only one who can set you free, and live as if you have already been set free.

Being Grateful Because It Is Already Mine

One of the simplest and most amazing things I have invested in was implementing gratitude and daily affirmations into my morning routine. This has created some amazing results. If you can remember, this was the one practice I gave up on because for a long time, I wasn't seeing any results. I am so glad I gave it a second attempt.

The mistakes I was making the first time around were: a) I didn't truly believe I was going to receive the results I was trying to manifest and had a lot of lingering doubts. I had to learn how to truly believe in what I was manifesting or else it would be a waste of time and waste of energy. I also had to mentally see myself with my desired results; b) I wasn't grateful in my affirmation. I later learned that saying "I have a lot of energy" just wasn't sufficient enough. In order to show God I truly believe it is already mine, I learned I needed to be as grateful as if I had already received it. I learned to thank God for what I had requested because He promises that if I pray and request for it, I should believe it is already mine. This is exactly how you should feel about your daily gratitudes and affirmations. My affirmation now looks and sounds a little like this now, "Thank you Lord for giving me so much energy."

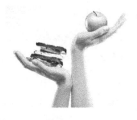

Chapter 5

I'm Feeling It All

*I*t has been so easy for us to get distracted and pay attention to only our outer world and our physical beings. Our society has taught us to pay attention to only our physical world, physical symptoms, and physical problems. We are never really taught that, in fact, we have negative emotions that can affect our health and affect us daily. We do not pay attention to our emotions, that is, until our emotions actually manifest into our physical world as physical pain. Sadly, if you visit a conventional doctor for your physical pain and symptoms, your emotions are never explored or discussed. The doctor would instead advise you to mask your physical pain or symptoms with prescription drugs, when in reality, all you probably needed was someone to talk you through your emotions. If you are lucky, your physician will refer you to a therapist, but many therapists also resort to prescribing anti-depressant drugs.

In order to help you make reasonable decisions, you must create emotional stability in your life because, by now, you know emotions can influence you to make the wrong choices or can lead you back to your never-ending binge cycles. We have been taught to hide our emotions. No one ever tells you that processing and taking time to feel your emotions is actually really beneficial. When you are finally able to process your negative emotions and release it to the Lord, you will no longer be held down by these negative emotions that you have been carrying around for far too long.

This chapter will help you identify negative emotions that have been trapped in your body and may have been holding you back from successfully beating your binge eating habit. You will discover how negative emotions can affect you physically and mentally. And finally, you will learn how to release these negative emotions, which will allow you to feel uplifted, rejuvenated, and ready to take on the world.

How Negative Emotions Impact Our Physical Health

Have you ever been so nervous that your stomach starts to feel uneasy and you start to get an upset stomach? For me, many times this would happen right before I had to get up in front of a group and complete a presentation. As soon as the presentation ends, my stress disappears, and my nerves go away. All of a sudden, my upset stomach seems to have also subsided. Even though heavily dismissed in our society, this is how emotions can impact you physically and mentally. Negative emotions typically derive from experiences, traumas, or beliefs that you have about yourself or the world. Not only can emotions talk you out of a healthy lifestyle, but emotions can also have an effect on your body that leads you to give in to binge eating.

Think about this, what if my upset stomach that was caused by nervousness did not subside even after I completed my presentation? Instead of checking to see if it was my nerves that caused my stomachache, we are trained to automatically assume that my stomachache was due to hunger pains. I will even start to talk to myself, trying to justify that after such a stressful presentation, in fact, I now deserve to treat myself out to my favorite buffet.

It has been previously thought that the mind would tell the body exactly what to do and how to feel, or that the mind and body were two separate entities. It is pretty clear now that the body has emotions that can also send information to the mind. Science has been teaching us that our body and mind has a mind/body connection that works together to communicate and support each other. In cases where negative emotions exist in the body, the mind/body connection can also deteriorate your health. For example, a large-scale epidemiological and medical study showed that employees with higher stressed jobs were twice as likely to develop metabolic syndrome, which leads to cardiovascular disease and type 2 diabetes. Another study completed by Psychosocial Research Laboratory at Stanford University determined that women with metastatic breast cancer who participated in group therapy along with their treatment plan had less pain, a better quality of life, and lived longer than their counterparts who did not participate in group therapy. Wow, what profound findings! We are learning that if we can support the negative emotions that run in our body and mind, we can improve our health and daily lives.

Even more amazing, neurotransmitters have been found in the immune system, which makes it possible for the body to communicate with the mind. This means that not only are our thoughts and feelings from the mind sending messages to our body, but any negative emotions that are trapped in the body can also affect both our physical health and mental health. Perhaps, the next time you experience a negative emotional experience, like bitterness or anger, you might think twice about processing your negative emotion right away, which will allow you the upper hand in controlling your binge eating.

Avoiding your negative emotions and holding onto negative emotions adds unnecessary stress to your body, and just isn't worth it. Continuous and constant stress will have your body constantly in flight or fight mode. Flight or fight mode puts your other daily bodily functions, such as digestion, on the back burner because your body thinks it needs to take care of this unnecessary stress from your negative emotions you are carrying around. Ultimately, over a long period of time, you will find your immune system, which is mainly housed in your digestive tract, becomes comprised. Unfortunately, the effects of being in fight or flight mode also means that your body regenerative capacity is also compromised. Most of our body's organs and tissues regenerate every few days, months, or years in order to keep our bodies running properly. When your regenerative capacity is reduced, you become prone to disease and illness.

Let's get you out of this rut so that your physical body and mental health can start operating properly. Getting out of the rut means that, with the right resources and guidance, you will need to take the time to process your feelings and emotions you have been bottling up and avoiding, and finally release these negative emotions. The process of releasing your negative emotions may be a hard and emotional one, but you will come out of it feeling awesome, uplifted, and relieved. My hope is that it will even help you relieve some physical pain and leverage your new healthier and binge-free lifestyle.

Emotional Eating

There is no doubt that emotional eating exists. It happens more often as we continue to have easy access to food. As our lives move in the direction of fast paced and instant gratification, where we want everything to be handed to us immediately, including the short-lived pleasure and satisfaction we get when we finally indulge in our favorite junk food, even at the cost of our health, we believe that these short-lived instant pleasures we get from our food will actually mend and heal our emotions.

Instead of taking your time to feel and sort out your negative emotions, you want to continue to avoid your emotions with simple instant distractions and pleasures. I encourage you to take the time to truly distinguish if you are truly physically hungry or just emotionally eating. Take the time to cook your food with love and gratitude. Fuel your body with real, nature-made food. Perhaps, when you experience longer lasting satisfaction from real food, you may be able to distinguish between emotional eating and true hunger.

In order to help you determine whether you are actually physically hungry or not, I suggest as soon as you feel hungry, you take a moment to reflect on your day. Has your day been stressful? Has it been filled with fear or nervousness? Have you spent your day mad at someone? If so, take a few minutes to release the negative emotion you felt today. All you have to do is verbally acknowledge the event or experience that caused you the negative emotion and verbally release the emotion that you experienced. Make sure to specifically mention your emotion. If you were angry, release anger; if you felt rejected, release rejection; if you felt guilty, release guilt, and so on. Once you release your negative emotion, you should start to feel better. If your physical symptoms or hunger remain, it may be true physical hunger you are experiencing. Eat a little to see if it makes you feel any better.

I often had to use this method to distinguish if I was truly hungry or not, whenever I found myself becoming angry or bitter at the people in my life who hurt me. Often times, I would feel hungry and discomfort around my pancreas. After I learned that the pancreas traps and holds feelings such as bitterness and disappointments, I knew it was in direct relation to the bitterness I felt towards the people in my life. The first time I released this particular emotion of bitterness, I could not believe what I was experiencing. My pancreas felt immediately better. I spent that whole night so thankful that my pancreas was finally starting to properly work while I listened to my pancreas gurgle every time I woke up. After this experience, I started using this method of releasing my negative emotions more often. Releasing your emotion is simple and sounds a little like this: *I acknowledge that my husband accusing me of not being able to control my temper made me bitter today. I release any feeling of bitterness and disappointments to you, Lord. Please continue to heal my body (or pancreas, if you know your specific body part or organ that has been affected by your negative emotion). Amen!*

It's Completely Okay to Feel Your Feelings

From as young as you can remember, you were taught to ignore or suppress your emotions. Remember your mom telling you not to cry anymore after you just had a painful fall because you are a big girl and big girls do not cry? Yep, I am also guilty of this. I tell my nieces and nephews at a very young age the same exact thing. I often had to remind myself that it is okay to process your feelings. In the midst of our busy lives, we prefer to ignore these feelings and emotions because these feelings show the world how vulnerable, weak, and emotional we are. Ignoring your feelings can only last so long until your emotions start manifesting into your physical world as either physical symptoms and pain, spiritual warfare, or even mental disorders.

You can try to avoid facing your emotions for as long as possible by distracting yourself with things of this world, such as shopping, drinking, technology, or even food. But your soul will remain empty for as long as it takes you to finally face your emotions. What might seem like a simple distraction or temporary relief may turn into a serious addiction. I am quite sure your binge eating cycle, to some extent, began because you had a negative belief about yourself or food, or you were hurt by someone you loved. In order to avoid being emotional, or perhaps because you didn't know how to process your feelings by yourself, you turned to food for comfort and distraction. But now you are finding yourself in a never-ending cycle of binge eating that you can no longer control.

I want to encourage you to feel your own feelings and emotions. Do what you need to do to release your negative emotion. Many times, you will find that releasing your negative emotion is simply acknowledging your feeling and verbally releasing it. Other times, you will find that you may need to cry it out, yell it out, or even pound it out of your system through physical activity, such as boxing. Do what you have to do to release your trapped negative emotions. Be proactive in releasing your negative emotions, and don't wait until physical symptoms show up before you pay attention to your feelings.

I will teach you a method of releasing your negative emotions. I would like to encourage you to release your negative emotions on a regular basis. Releasing your negative emotions is an on-going process. Even though we all wish that we can just release all of our negative emotions in one session, life just doesn't work like that. You may need a few sessions to release your past negative emotions that have been built up. Once all of your past negative emotions are released, life is still going to throw your way experiences and traumas that will stir up a lot of emotions. Your job is to process and release those negative emotions you encounter as soon as possible. This will help you leverage your binge eating habit because you won't be carrying around unneeded negative emotions that will have you making rash, undesirable decisions.

As you start releasing your emotions, you will learn that you are a unique person who has experienced different events and traumas that have affected you. This means that you may have layers upon layers of negative emotions that need to be released. Most of my clients have expressed to me that taking the extra time to discuss and sort out their emotions and emotional experiences with me was much needed and gave them such a soothing and uplifting session. Take your time in feeling and releasing each emotion. It's going to be a process. Your body will tell you when you are ready to release the next emotion. Don't rush it; it's a lifestyle change. You have the rest of your life to release your trapped negative emotions. You may even find yourself having to release the same emotion many times, when you find yourself experiencing the same emotion over and over throughout your life.

What Causes Trapped Negative Emotions?

There are many negative emotions that we experience in our lifetime due to experiences and traumas we go through or beliefs we have about ourselves or the world. We all have different life experiences and also have different perspective of the same exact event. Even if you and I attended the same exact event, your perception and the emotions you experience may be totally different from mine. Through your life experiences and perceptions, you encounter negative emotions that can become trapped inside of you, also known as trapped negative emotions. When you do not take the time to process or feel your emotions and release these negative emotions, these negative emotions can affect you adversely, impacting you mentally, physically, and emotionally. As you have learned in quantum physics, energy is communicated through our feelings. Ultimately what this means is that feelings and emotions are energy. We can feel our emotions throughout our body because energy travels and vibrates in and around us. Releasing negative emotions helps you to create a stabilized emotional state and ensures that your environment is filled with only positive energy.

Some of our trapped negative emotions can be easily identified. These trapped negative emotions are caused by experiences and traumas that you can recall. These are the negative emotions you can easily identify and release. However, I want you to know that there are some trapped negative emotions that may have affected you but have gone unnoticed, even if you can remember the event. For example, let's say you got into an argument with your brother. You remember this argument caused you to experience bitterness that may have caused a trapped emotion of bitterness, but you may not have noticed that this same exact argument caused a trap emotion of guilt. These unnoticed, trapped negative emotions, once discovered, also need to be addressed and released.

A good example of a trapped negative emotion is the day your parents announced to you and your brothers that they were getting a divorce. On that particular day, you felt that everything was your fault, including their decision to get divorced, and you were filled with guilt. You also felt abandoned. You were so worried about how you and your brothers would go on, and most importantly, who would be taking care of your two younger brothers. You felt helpless. You thought there was something you could do to change their mind, but really nothing could be done. The divorce was done and final. This one event may have caused you more than one trapped negative emotion, which must be released when your body is ready to release them.

There are other trapped negative emotions that happen without your conscious knowledge, or maybe you just can't recall the event that caused the trapped negative emotion. These unknown trapped negative emotions can be inherited from your parents and ancestors just like you can inherit your hair color, height, and skin color from them. Trapped negative emotions can be inherited when you were in your mother's womb, even before you were born. Some of the negative emotions that were felt by your mother while you were in her womb can remain with you throughout your life. These negative emotions that are unknown still have the ability to affect your physical body and mental health, just like an easily identifiable emotion can affect you adversely. Even if you are not aware or cannot identify these negative emotions that may be holding you back, the method I teach you will help you identify and discover these unknown trapped negative emotions so that you can release them.

A client of mine, Dawn, came to me because whenever she would give in to her binge eating cycles, she was always feeling overwhelmingly unworthy and unwanted. As you will also learn how to do, we were able to discover that even though Dawn grew up with a very happy family with her mom, her step-father, and her two half-sisters, her mom's life before meeting her step-father has caused Dawn to feel unworthy and unwanted. Dawn's biological father, according to her mother, was always very verbally and physically abusive. He always made her mother feel unwanted and unworthy, even when she was pregnant with Dawn. We found out that these emotions that Dawn had never experienced directly had a huge impact on her life today.

Releasing Your Identified Trapped Negative Emotions

Let me introduce you to the sway test. This method was introduced to me by my NTP mentor. I later learned the details of this method by a great doctor, Dr. Bradley Nelson. This test will help confirm any trapped negative emotions you have and will help you identify any trapped negative emotions you may not be aware of. The sway test communicates with your subconscious mind to identify negative emotions that are linked to experiences and traumas that caused them. There is a total of three steps that need to be taken. Once you can identify your trapped negative emotions, I will teach you how to go ahead and release those negative emotions.

Step 1: Testing your baseline

To get started with the sway test, you want to establish a baseline. This will help you to determine if your subconscious mind is ready to communicate with you. The easiest way to do this is to make sure you are relaxed. Stand with your eyes closed and your feet shoulder width apart, in a quiet room free from distractions and noises. Make sure you are standing comfortably balanced. All questions or statements should be made out loud. You want to test your baseline by first making a true statement and then making a false statement. Subconsciously, your body will sway forward to all statements that are true, and sway backward to all statements that are false. This is your subconscious mind communicating with you. Speaking out loud, use this true statement to test your baseline: "My name is (state your real name)." Your body should have swayed forward. Use this false statement to test your baseline: "My name is (make up a name that is not yours)." Your body should have swayed backward. Test a few other true and false statements. Once you have established your baseline, where your body is swaying forward according to your true statements and backward to your false statements, you are ready to start discovering your trapped negative emotions.

If, for some reason, you are cannot find your baseline, which means your body is not swaying forward when you are making a true statement and your body does not sway backward when you are making a false statement, you may want to take a break. Take a few deep breaths, drink some water, get refocused, make sure to be relaxed and forget about being in control. Try testing your baseline over again.

Step 2: Determine if you have any trapped negative emotions
Once you have successfully tested your baseline, use the sway test to determine if you have any trapped negative emotions that need to be released. Start by making this statement "Do I have a trapped emotion that can be released at this moment?" If you sway forward that means your trapped negative emotion is ready to be released. If you sway backward, even though unlikely, this may mean you do not have any trapped negative emotions, or it may mean a trapped negative emotion exists, but is not yet ready to be released. Remember, take your time.

Listen to your body. It's going to be a process. Do not force a release of your trapped emotion.

Step 3: Determine the specific negative emotion you need to release

In this next step, you will use the emotions list I have included in the *Negative Emotions Chart* to determine your specific trapped negative emotion (see Appendix B). Your subconscious mind is aware of trapped negative emotions that need to be release, even

Negative Emotions Chart			
	Column A	Column B	Column C
Row 1	Abandoned Abused Anger Anxiety Ashamed	Empty Envious Exposed Failure Fearful	Mocked Nervous Powerless Pride Rejected
Row 2	Attacked Betrayed Bitter Blame Broken-Hearted	Frustrated Grief Guilty Harrassed Hated	Resentment Sadness Shameful Terror Trapped
Row 3	Burdened Condemned Conflicted Criticized Decieved	Helpless Hopelessness Humiliated Hurt Insulted	Vulnerable Undersirable Worthless Worry Trapped
Row 4	Depressed Desperate Disappointed Disgust Embarassed	Intimdated Insecure Isolated Manipulated Mistreated	Violated Vulnerable Undersirable Used Worthless

without reading the emotions on this list. You can—but do not need to—read over the chart before getting started.

You need to determine if your trapped negative emotion is listed on the Negative Emotions Chart. Using the sway test, ask, "Is this trapped emotion listed in Column A?" Continue to ask, "Is this trapped emotion listed in Column B?" "Is this trapped emotion listed in Column C?" Keep asking until your body sways forward to a specific column. Keep in mind that you may have more than one trapped negative emotion. Work on releasing one emotion at a time. If your subconscious mind

Negative Emotions Chart		
	Column A	Column B	Column C
Row 1	Abandoned Abused Anger Anxiety Ashamed	Empty Envious Exposed Failure Fearful	Mocked Nervous Powerless Pride Rejected
Row 2	Attacked Betrayed Bitter Blame Broken-Hearted	Frustrated Grief Guilty Harrassed Hated	Resentment Sadness Shameful Terror Trapped
Row 3	Burdened Condemned Conflicted Criticized Decieved	Helpless Hopelessness Humiliated Hurt Insulted	Vulnerable Undersirable Worthless Worry Trapped
Row 4	Depressed Desperate Disappointed Disgust Embarassed	Intimdated Insecure Isolated Manipulated Mistreated	Violated Vulnerable Undersirable Used Worthless

happens to tell you that you have trapped negative emotions on more than one column, take a deep breath and ask God to show you the truth, and try again until you can pinpoint only one column.

Let's pretend you swayed forward when you asked if your trapped negative emotion is in Column B. Your next step is to keep narrowing down your negative emotions. You now want to figure out which row under Column B your trapped negative emotion is in, and ask, "Is this trapped emotion listed in Row 1?" "Is this trapped emotion listed in Row 2?" and so on.

Negative Emotions Chart			
	Column A	Column B	Column C
Row 1	Abandoned Abused Anger Anxiety Ashamed	Empty Envious Exposed Failure Fearful	Mocked Nervous Powerless Pride Rejected
Row 2	Attacked Betrayed Bitter Blame Broken-Hearted	Frustrated Grief Guilty Harrassed Hated	Resentment Sadness Shameful Terror Trapped
Row 3	Burdened Condemned Conflicted Criticized Decieved	Helpless Hopelessness Humiliated Hurt Insulted	Vulnerable Undersirable Worthless Worry Trapped
Row 4	Depressed Desperate Disappointed Disgust Embarassed	Intimdated Insecure Isolated Manipulated Mistreated	Violated Vulnerable Undersirable Used Worthless

By the time you have determined which row your emotion is in, you should have narrowed your trapped negative emotion to only five possible emotions that need to be released. The last step in identifying your specific trapped negative emotion is to ask which one of these five emotions is your trapped emotion. Let's say you swayed forward to Row 2. You want to go through each emotion individually in Row 2, Column B to pinpoint the one correct trapped emotion. Start by asking, "Is this trapped emotion frustration?" Continue to ask if this trapped emotion is grief, guilt, harassment, or hatred. Your body should sway forward and answer "yes" to one of these five emotions.

For the sake of this next illustration, let's say your trapped negative emotion was guilt.

Releasing your negative emotion is simple.

Step 1 of releasing your negative emotions:
Accept the emotion that has been trapped. Take a moment to feel the emotion. If you can recall the event or trauma that caused this negative emotion to be trapped, take some time to acknowledge the event or experience that caused the trapped negative emotion.

Remember that these trapped negative emotions became stuck because you never got the chance to feel and process your emotions.

This might be a very emotional experiment. If you need to, feel free to cry it out, scream, or even stomp it out.

Step 2 of releasing your emotion:
Say this short, powerful prayer to help you release your trapped negative emotion:

> *Dear Lord,*
>
> *Thank You for showing me my trapped emotion of guilt (name your specific trapped emotion). I release this trapped emotion of guilt (name your specific trapped emotion). I forgive myself for carrying around this emotion. I forgive (list the people who were involved in the event that happened to cause this trapped emotion, if known) my mom and dad for causing this emotion to be trapped when they got divorced. I release this emotion of guilt to you. Please fill me with Your peace and continue to give me a spirit of power, love, and self-control.*
>
> *Amen!*

One of my clients, Susan, came to me because she had periodic chest pain that came and went. But when they came, she felt like her heart was going to jump out of her chest. By the time she started working with me, she had already gone to the emergency room, a check-up with her primary, and even to see a cardiologist, but nothing could be found or detected. She was always in decently good health and so she was convinced it was more than physical. As I got to know her and her story, she was able to recall, recently in the last year or so, that she experienced a lot of disappointments with her husband not living up to her expectations. To add on top of that, her teenage daughter, who was always a good kid, recently started dating, lying to her, and even started to slack off with her school work on purpose. As we started releasing these feelings, she discovered that she was, in fact, holding in a lot of negative emotions of betrayal, disappointment, and heartbreak. She reported to me a week later that, in addition to taking her ibuprofen, which she had been taking for a while, her chest pain seemed to have slowly disappeared. She believes it was this exercise that helped her identify her negative emotions and eliminate her chest pain because ibuprofen was only really good at masking her chest pain in the past. Susan even came to the point where she realized she had to forgive her husband and daughter, and keep moving forward, even if life doesn't go exactly the way she hoped for.

Deeper Explorations

Sometimes your subconscious mind may want to give you more information about your trapped negative emotion. If you dig deeper, your subconscious mind may tell you when this emotion became trapped, and what experience or trauma caused this emotion to be trapped. Other times, all you may discover is the specific emotion and nothing about how that trapped emotion came about.

In order to dig deeper, you will want to ask, "Is there anything else I should know about my emotion of guilt (name negative emotion) that has been trapped?" If not, go ahead and release it.

In order to dig deeper, you want to ask when this emotion became trapped. Narrow down the when by determining your approximate age. Start by asking, "Did this emotion become trapped before I turned eleven years old?" If yes, go ahead and continue to narrow down your approximate age. Close this age gap down by asking, "Did this emotion become trapped after I turned five?" If yes, continue to ask, "Did this emotion become trapped when I was six years old?" Continue to ask until you get a forward sway to see whether the emotion became trapped when you were seven years old, eight years old, nine years old and so on. Many times, you might get an approximate age, for example between the ages of nine and ten.

Once you know that you were approximately nine to ten years old when this emotion became trapped, you want to start thinking of possible events that happened when you were nine to ten years old that might have caused this trapped emotion. For example, if you recall that your parents got divorced right after your tenth birthday, you would want to ask, "Did this emotion become trapped after my tenth birthday?" If yes, you are now more certain it was your parent's divorce that caused this trapped negative emotion. You would then want to ask if this emotion became trapped due to your parent's divorce. Once you have reached this point of discovery, you will want to take time to feel the emotion, acknowledge the event, and release this emotion.

There may be times when you just can't pinpoint the specific event that caused this trapped negative emotion. Another option to help you dig deeper is to try and determine who was involved in the event or trauma that caused this trapped negative emotion. After narrowing down your age, as we did above, you will want to ask if people who were in your life at that time were involved in creating your trapped emotion. For example, if you had no possible idea your emotion became trapped because of your parent's divorce, but you do know that this guilt became trapped when you were nine to ten years old, you would want to go through all the possible people that were involved in your life when you were nine to ten years old. You would ask questions like, "Was it a family member that caused this trapped emotion?" If yes, you will want to go through your list of family members that were in your life at the time. Ask, "Was it my mom who caused this trapped emotion?" If for some reason you discovered it was not your family that caused your trapped negative emotion, you can dig deeper by asking if other people in your life might have caused your trapped emotion, like your friends, your teacher, or your doctor. Once you can determine who was involved, it will hopefully help you further determine the event that caused this trapped negative emotion. If possible, confirm the event that caused your trapped negative emotion based on the person who was involved in causing your trapped negative emotion, and release that emotion.

Continue this same process of releasing your negative emotions when you feel the need to find emotional stability in your life. My hope is that you will learn to enjoy the process. Your body and soul will thank you. You will learn to love the feeling of being rejuvenated, peaceful, and uplifted after releasing your negative emotions. In order to continue living a peaceful life after releasing each emotion, try your best to live in the present. Living in the past will cause you to become depressed, as you continue to dwell on past trauma and hurtful events. There is nothing you can do about the past. Focusing on the future will cause you to become anxious. You will spend unnecessary energy on things you cannot control. You will even spend wasted time on things that may never even happen. Be happy; stay present!

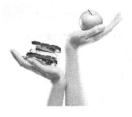

Chapter 6

Environmental Support System

*H*ave you ever committed to starting a healthier lifestyle, but everywhere you look there's temptations? You open your kitchen cabinet, and there's a chocolate bar staring at you. You open your refrigerator, and those thick slices of bacon are calling your name. You go to your freezer, and your favorite bucket of ice cream has been waiting for you all day. You can see how easy it is to get distracted and resort back to your binge eating cycle when you are always surrounded by your favorite junk food.

Of course, you may not be able to control all aspects of your life because you may be living or working with others who are not yet on a journey to a healthier lifestyle. Either way, we want to set you up for success. Setting yourself up for success is the best thing you can proactively do. Using the concepts and techniques you just learned in the last few chapters, I want you to build environments both at home and work, which will support you in reaching your goal.

A Homey Environment

You probably know that having a support system in place will better set you up for success. My goal is to ensure you do have a strong support system in place so that you can successfully break free from binge eating. When you have someone who is constantly wondering how you are doing, how your healthier lifestyle is treating you, you are prone to stick to your goals. We tend to want to please the people we care about and love, and are less likely to fail them. We want to be able to deliver on our commitments, even our verbal commitments.

Think about this, if you were thinking about planning a surprise birthday party for your mother, and if you discussed this party with your two younger brothers, you are more likely to commit to throwing this birthday party. If you planned this party by yourself without telling anyone, you can choose to change your mind at any time and even decide at the last minute not to throw her a surprise birthday party. But once your brothers know you are planning a party, you now have them excited and they probably want to be involved in the entire planning process. They are expecting you to commit to throwing this surprise birthday party for your mother, making it less likely for you to back out, unless you had a true last-minute emergency.

I would encourage you to get yourself an accountability partner. This does not mean tell everyone your goals. It means you need to pick one or two trusted friends or family members that you know will help get you back on track and keep pushing you forward. This person should be someone who will be honest and respectful towards you. They will let you know when you need to get back on track, help you get back on track, and even become your support system when you need someone to keep you away from giving into your cravings and temptations.

Not only should you get yourself an accountability partner, but you should also get your significant other on the same page as you. You need to create an environment at home that is supportive. Besides, most of your time is either spent at home or work, and you need to create an environment that helps you to leverage breaking your habit of binge eating, and it starts with creating a supportive environment at home.

This doesn't exactly mean he has to eat what you are eating because maybe he just isn't ready to eat healthier or maybe he doesn't have to be set free of binge eating. But this does mean that he should understand your goals for yourself. Communicating with your significant other your goals will leverage him to be more supportive. You will find he will become more supportive in encouraging you to buy the nutrient-filled food you need to accomplish your goals, even if it means double the cost for food. You will get the mental and verbal support you need from him. The second he notices changes in you, he will encourage you to keep going or even let you know when he has noticed how your waist is getting slimmer and a bit more defined. Once he starts to see your shift in mood and energy, the people you love, including your significant other, will start to enjoy being around you more as you are happy and uplifted. Once your significant other sees enough change in you and your habits, he might even jump on the healthy lifestyle with you, engage in physical activities with you, or engage in meal prepping with you.

Getting your significant other on the same page as you means you are, most importantly, getting more time for self-care. You will notice that if you have to take a little more time than usual for yourself to detox, rejuvenate, or for self-care, he becomes more supportive and understanding. Remember, communication is the key to getting the support you need to achieve the goal you have been wanting.

Amy, one of my clients, was always the quiet and reserved one in her relationship with her husband. Most times, she felt as if she did not know how to express her feelings, desires, and plans for starting a healthier lifestyle to her husband. Day in and day out, she would inform her husband that tomorrow she was going to stop eating uncontrollably. In our third session, I sat down with her and made it clear to her that clearly communicating with her husband was the only way he was ever going to support her or at least slightly understand her. We sat down and looked at her goal of finally taking control of her binge eating habit. We made a list of the benefits she would experience once she was binge-free. She was going to share these benefits with her husband. Together, we set boundaries and guidelines that she felt comfortable expressing to her husband to ensure they were both on the same page and so she could get all the support she would need. To my surprise, a few weeks later, she expressed to me how grateful she was to have that session with me. It made such a difference in how her husband approached her. He was so much more supportive than before, and he even seemed to understand her more when she needed just a little more time for herself. He noticed she was more energized and definitely enjoyed this new found energy.

Actually Love the People You Work With

I get it. You are at the peak of your career. You have been able to move up your desired career ladder with not much effort. You are now finally settling into your new position. It's been about nine months since you got promoted into your current position. Things seemed to be going smoothly, and you have had so much motivation. That is, up until this point. You are beginning to realize that, not only have you been so stressed and busy with work, but your binge eating cycle is doing nothing but leading you into depression. You can't even focus on work anymore, and have somehow lost your motivation. Your binge eating cycle is leaving you exhausted, and you are just going through the motions in life. You also haven't been in the best health lately. Even though you have always been heavier set, more recently your physical symptoms have gotten worse. Your stomach pains are showing up more consistently when you eat now, after eating you feel so bloated, and your muscles seem to cramp and ache whenever they feel like it. Just in the last month, you started feeling this tingling feeling when you pee and just in the last two weeks, when you pee it's just downright painful. Everything seems to be falling apart. Even though you are still able to keep up at work as of now, with things falling apart at this rate, you are now worried that your job performance might also reflect how horribly you feel these days.

The first thing you need to do is to look at your environment at work and determine which stress factors you can reduce. Remember, stress is an emotion and it can cause rash decisions and cause unnecessary physical and mental illnesses. Is it that your workload is too much or too stressful? Or is it that the people around you at work are just impossible to work with? Whatever it is that is stressing you out, your goal is to reduce it as much as you can. You can use what you have learned in quantum physics to create an environment and workload that is supportive to you and the desired life you want.

Let's say, for example, your workload and work projects are actually very stressful and demanding. Instead of using that energy you spend stressing over your workload and project, use that energy to meditate and rehearse your workload and your projects. Meditating on your workload will allow you to know exactly what you need to do to complete your projects, because of course, you have completed these same projects many times before in your head. Rehearse all the steps you need to take in order to complete your project. Meditate on how easy it was to complete your project because everything you needed to complete your project was readily available. Imagine confidently presenting the end result to your manager and the rest of your team. You come out of this project with a smile on your face and extremely satisfied about how everything went.

Your manager meets you outside of the conference room after your presentation and even congratulates and tells you how awesome your presentation went. Continue to rehearse this daily until you actually successfully complete your project with less stress. You got this because you have done it so many times in your mind!

You can use the same method to get over that one co-worker who seems to always be looking over your shoulder at everything you do, who seems to always be gossiping about one person or another, and who always has an attitude about everything and anything that does not go her way. You are going to want to use meditation to rehearse your everyday interaction with her, and instead of reacting the same way, you want to react differently. In your meditation sessions, the next time you see yourself in the lunchroom with her and once again she is angry or irritated about something, instead of rolling your eyes and ignoring her, you want to approach her differently. Imagine walking up to her, with an intent to hear why she is so stressed out or angry, and try to understand her perspective. Imagine having a full conversation with her that actually opens up your own perspective. You walk away from that conversation feeling quite satisfied that both of you are actually on the same page and were actually able to release some of the same frustrations. The next time you actually see her in the lunchroom, you want to approach her exactly how you did in your meditation session. You might even find that you both are facing the same problem and might be able to approach your manager with similar solutions to your problems. She might even become a close co-worker because you had so much more in common than you previously thought, and even if you don't become closer, you can at least exist in the same space civilly.

Finding Your Day Time Focus

Have you noticed that part of the reason you are so stressed about work is that you actually bring it home with you? Even after you just finished an eight- to ten-hour workday, you are still thinking about work. You may or may not have physically brought home your work, but your mind is constantly thinking about it. Keep in mind that you must be in the present moment to be at peace. Remind yourself not to get caught up in anxiousness or fear. Even if you are up stressing and thinking about work, you probably can't do anything about your work project that is actually at work. Most nights you even find yourself tossing and turning in bed because you are thinking and stressing about work. Yes, you should definitely take the time to meditate about your work projects, but meditation should take no longer than ten to fifteen minutes. Meditation shouldn't be keeping you anxious and up at night. Besides, your goal in meditating is to make your workload easier, not more stressful.

Keep in mind that as hard as you have worked to get to where you are, even if you have the best relationship with your managers, or you love your company to the moon and back, you are replaceable. Your company will replace you as soon as you are unable to work due to a physical or mental illness, or even worse—God forbid—you can easily be replaced if something horrible were to happen to you. Your job will easily replace you, but what you cannot replace are you and your health. Keep you and your health at the top of your priority list—not your work. Do what you can and leave the rest at work.

I had to learn the hard way that work sure isn't worth staying up for. Staying up thinking about work not only takes away from your beauty sleep, but also take away from both your mental and physical health. When you miss out on sleep, you are also missing out on a lot of your body's regenerative capacity, which leads to an imbalance of your much-needed bodily hormones and chemicals. Over a period of time, your body and mental health will deteriorate.

Are you wondering why you haven't been able to focus lately? Wondering why you have been so irritable and have been feeling so emotionally unstable? If you are staying up late thinking about work, deprivation of sleep is probably one of your main contributing factors! Oh yes, we don't want to forget your physical symptoms that have been showing up, such as your stomach pain and feeling bloated—those can directly correlate to your lack of sleep. Lack of sleep weakens your digestive and immune systems because certain chemicals and proteins, like cykotines, which are found in your immune system, will not be able to produce the amount your body needs. Cykotines are released during sleep and need to increase in order to help fight viruses and inflammation, but the proper amount cannot be released if you are lacking sleep.

I had a client, Carla, who came to me desperately wanting to get a full night's sleep. She had gotten to the point where she realized that no matter how many hours she spent tossing and turning every night over work, there was nothing positive that came out of staying up all night. She felt drained and even started noticing dark circles appearing under her eyes just six months into this new job she recently got promoted to. She informed me she had tried everything she could think of to try and help her sleep, but was not successful. Unfortunately, for her, she probably made staying up a habit for such a long time that her body thought it was normal. I gave her something to try that I consistently use now because I also used to stay up all night thinking about work. I informed her that perhaps her tossing and turning, like it was for me, was a sign that God wanted to talk to her and to spend some time with her. It was not a time He wanted her to use to stay up and worry about work, but just a time to get a little conversation in with her. I advised her that next time she was up tossing and turning, she should invite the Lord in for a conversation. It's super easy. All she needed to say was "Lord, I invite you in to talk to me. Please open my heart and allow me to hear anything you need me to hear." Carla tried it for a while before she was able to report anything to me. She found it easier to fall asleep the first two weeks and thought that might have just been a coincidence that her sleep patterns were getting better because her eating habit was also getting better. About the third week, she noticed she started hearing that small, still voice that believers typically experience as God speaking. That small, still voice gave her some revelations and answers to her prayers, but most importantly, it gave her peace; she was finally able to get in several full nights of sleep.

Do Not Allow Work to Take the Place of God

As humans, we strive so hard toward securing our financial futures and reaching our financial goals. We start as young as four years old and work for many, many years just so we make a living. Even though we should reach for the stars and dream big dreams, making a living is really all we should be aiming for, especially if it is at the cost of your own health. I believe that before you decide to put your health on the back burner, all you should be really aiming for is making enough money so that you and your family can feel comfortable and be able to enjoy some time together. We are so consumed with our worldly desires that we slave day in and out just to be able to purchase everything we could possibly think of. Our goal of getting the latest gadget or the best of everything is simply driving us to allow money to control us, and sadly driving us faster to a diseased body than ever before.

Most of us don't realize how important it is to be proactive in taking care of ourselves, whether that's taking time to rejuvenate or taking control of your binge eating habit before too much damage is done. Don't wait until it is too late. Many times, you completely avoid all the physical, emotional, and even mental symptoms that your body has been giving you as hints for years, such as stomach pain, not being able to focus, or emotional instability. You continue to go through the motions of life, making as much money as you possibly can, until one day you are admitted into the emergency room with unbearable stomach pain, only to find out you have a chronic disease, such as cancer or diabetes. For many of us, only then will our life flash before our eyes. At this moment, money is nothing more than a piece of paper. A piece of paper that you have been chasing all your life at the cost of your health. Don't let it be that only when you are hit with a chronic or deathly illness, you finally realize that money is worthless compared to something priceless, like good health. Even if you are lucky enough to get a second chance at life and come out of the hospital with a chronic disease, you have already caused so much damage to your body that even though possible, it would be difficult to get back to where you once were, healthy and free.

I cannot emphasize how important it is to take time for yourself and your health so that you can live a long life, filled with energy and vitality. Do not allow work to become an idol. Just like food can become an idol, so can work. Without realizing it, we all at one point or another have allowed work to become an idol of ours. You have allowed work to become an idol when you think about work day and night, you let it control you, and give it more value than anything else. I also used to make an idol out of work, but I found out that it was ruining my health and was unsupportive of my new binge-free lifestyle. I had to learn how to do the best I could at work, and allow God to become my idol, and take my stress away from me. I hope you can do the same for your sake.

Finding God's Purpose in Your Line of Work

In whatever line of work you are in, wherever your professional career lies, my hope is that you use your line of work and skills to complete your purpose that God has for you. Use your line of work to represent God and introduce people you come in contact with to God and His truth. What is His truth? His truth is that He loves you and that He sent his only son to die on the cross for your sins. His truth is that you are His daughter and deserve all that is wonderful. His truth is embedded in each and every one of our stories, including yours. Exposing God and His truth doesn't have to be forced or even salesy, connect people with God through your story. Be an example of the grace and peace God gives us, be a living example of God's miracles. God wants you to show others how He has changed you. Make the connection! You will soon understand that more people than you can imagine are struggling in similar situations and can be inspired by your story.

Christian-based companies are growing everywhere because they have the same desire to introduce everyone they come in contact with, both believers and non-believers, to God. They want to ensure their business, work, and skills are used as an expression of worship to God. There are restaurants, coffee shops, and even wedding dress companies that are centered around God. Your line of work doesn't even have to be business or company, there are stay-at-home moms, teachers, and social workers making a difference in other people's lives. You, too, can do the same.

Approaching someone about God doesn't have to be intimidating or difficult. I still use this method often before introducing people to God. Even though it should come more naturally, I am only human and am taking it one day at a time. Pray about a specific person before approaching them. Let God know you would like for God to work in their heart before you approach them. Get to know them like you have done in the past with anyone you first meet. Introduce them to God through your story. Ask them to come to church, your prayer circle, or even a bible study that you believe will help them in sorting out their own problems. Remind them of special

Christian-based events that might interest them, like women-based conferences or even Christian concerts. Do your part, let go, and let God. Only God can truly change their heart.

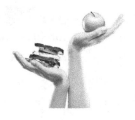

Chapter 7

Fueling My Body

*Y*ay! You are finally here! You have built yourself a strong enough foundation. I am confident that this foundation will hold you up when you are faced with temptations and cravings. Now, let's build you an even stronger foundation by giving you all the knowledge and resources you will need to succeed nutritionally. I want you to know exactly what you need to fuel your body with.

What We Have Been Taught

Society and government agencies have always had a huge influence on us, on the way we dress, think, and even what we eat. Society even impacts the way we think about food and our health.

Our society has shifted from an agricultural world to a money-making world, where most of the products in our grocery stores are genetically modified or heavily fertilized. Besides the produce aisle, most of us know nothing about what is actually in our food and what we are actually feeding our bodies, but yet we find it acceptable, as a society, to feed our future generations these unknown products, which we call food. Certain known junk food, like Oreos and soda, are now even labeled as organic. Nothing is organic about Oreos or soda besides being organically created in a chemistry lab.

Our society has gone from health care to managed care. Our doctors and healthcare corporations are no longer interested in truly educating their patients so they can truly take care of themselves. The word "doctor" derives from the Latin word for "teacher." Our healthcare system has moved so far away from this module of educating and teaching their patients about how to be proactive in taking control of their health or how to completely rid themselves of their illnesses. The healthcare system is more interested in masking the symptoms of their patients. The goal of our healthcare system should be to focus on finding the root cause of each illness so that patients do not have to continually visit their doctor's office as their masked symptoms reappear or additional symptoms show up. But of course, finding the solution to the root cause of each illness just won't bring in enough income. Our healthcare system has pulled itself so far away that most of the root causes of chronic illnesses we face today are still unknown. Instead, we blame genetics for these illnesses. This leads patients to think that there is nothing they can do or change to influence and take control of their own health.

Our society and governmental agencies have failed us in their quest to make money. The governments recommended our society to accept the Standard American Diet (SAD) for decades, while they continue to grow the dairy and junk food corporations. As a society, we are now in such a frantic state of poor health, so much so that we are constantly looking for the next fad diet that will hopefully work, to help us live healthier lives. Our society is not only confused about the state of our health, but to add fuel to the fire, with food so readily available, we are finding social gatherings and family functions filled with as much junk food and processed food as possible. These readily available junk food and processed foods open the door for mindless eating instead of using food for what it was intended for, which is fueling our body.

A Shift in Perspective

It is obvious our old perspectives and ways of thinking just don't work. We have been living out these old ways of thinking for years, even decades. When things haven't been working, perhaps, we should try something different. We are creatures of habit and new things may seem scary, but nothing is scarier than risking your own health and life to something that has proven not to work.

It's similar to the way we conduct things in our everyday life. If you were part of a team that implemented a new process at work, and this new process failed your clients over and over, there is no way that your company would allow you to continue to implement it. It just doesn't work like that. So, the question now is, "Why are you allowing our society's perspective and knowledge determine your health and your quality of life?"

Let me prove it to you.

The United States Department of Agriculture's Agriculture and Food Statistics report shows that small agricultural family farms started to decline in 1935. In 2012, there were only two million small family farms across America, versus six million in 1935. What this means is that the decline in small family farms led to an increase in big corporate farms. Big corporate farms brought along with them a mass growth of genetically modified food and a massive amount of fertilizer used to grow our foods. Small family farms typically meant more organic farming. This also meant more physical activity. Growing your own garden takes some pretty intense work. Why is it that our society is telling us that it is perfectly okay to poison us with chemicals and genetically modified food? Even more personally, why are you allowing yourself to poison your body?

Like me, you have probably jumped on the well-known Atkin's version of the keto diet, which introduced lowering your carbohydrate intake, including limiting most sources of nutritious, fiber-filled vegetables and fruits. I am not saying the keto diet doesn't work, but I am saying that suggesting I can eat an unlimited amount of animal protein, including animal fat, is absurd. Have you ever heard someone approach you and say something like, "I have been on this keto diet. It's been amazing. I can eat all the bacon I want and still lose weight?" I have to admit, I have been guilty of that. This is where we are making a huge mistake. Our society has us focusing on losing weight and not getting healthy. The perspective we are used to is completely wrong. We should be focusing on health first and not weight loss.

This last example will give you a better understanding of our current health management system that a lot of people seem to be perfectly content with. Even though heart disease continues to increase, the mortality rate due to heart disease has decreased. The decrease is probably due to better technology and treatment. Keeping us alive longer is great, but our goal as a society should not just to keep us living longer, but also living a better quality of life as we age. Living longer with great quality is achievable; many healthy societies have done it and so can we.

Let's look at smoking. Smoking is a major contributor to heart disease. Over the past fifteen years, smoking has decreased by twenty percent in the US, but why is it that heart disease continues to increase? There is only one other major contributor I can think of that contributes to the increase in heart disease—our food. While smoking has decreased, obesity rates continue to increase and have increased by forty-eight percent in the last fifteen years. Body mass index (BMI) and diabetes contribute to heart disease; our food choices also affect our BMI and the development of diabetes. We have to do better as a society when fueling our bodies; and more importantly, we have to decide on an individual basis that we can no longer continue to feed our bodies processed and diseased food.

I am going to encourage you to also take on a new way of thinking with your new way of living. I encourage you to take a stance for your own health and well-being. Start thinking about what you are really putting into your body and what you are fueling your body with. What worked best for me was every time I put something in my mouth, I quickly evaluated whether or not this food would glorify God and the temple He gave me.

Don't let your previous knowledge of what we have been taught all our lives about genetics limit your future and your health. Epigenetics, a more recent phenomenon, is a study of how genes are expressed. Epigenetics states that our environment has the ability to turn on and off genes. This means that our genes do not exactly determine or dictate the destiny of our health. Have you ever heard someone say to you, "I now have diabetes. It's genetics. There is nothing I can do about it." Wrong! Chronic diseases like diabetes and cancer can be avoided and, in some cases, even reversed. Remember, it is not only our genes that control our health but also our environmental factors. Get this, unlike we have been taught all of our lives, only five to ten percent of diseases, like certain cancers, can be attributed to hereditary genes. Did you hear that?! Only five to ten percent of diseases can be attributed to hereditary genes! This means that at least ninety percent of our health can be influenced by our environmental factors. With this in mind, we can finally stop blaming genetics and start taking control of our health.

I advise you to start your new way of thinking and start living your best life today. Don't plan for a cheat day even though we all know it happens. I once heard that, similar to a person going in for Alcoholics Anonymous (AA) treatment to help their alcohol addiction, the best method to getting them out of addiction is to have them go all in. All in, meaning go cold turkey. No cheating. This is the best way to get you going.

It's just a jump start to your new lifestyle, once you get the hang of controlling your binge eating, you can give yourself some leeway.

With so many fad diets out there, I would suggest you not stick to a specific nutritional plan. Don't even stick to one label, like vegan or vegetarian. Eat a variety of nature made food. Don't be limited by a label. Listen to your body. You and your body know best. Do not let a label or specific diet define your success. Sometimes when you focus too much on a specific label or diet, it starts to limit you because you will start to focus on the wrong details, such as counting calories or counting carbs versus actually getting healthy.

> *"Study the habits of the people you want to be like and then imitate them. If they are succeeding, they must be doing something right."*
> **– Dave Ramsey**

As Dave Ramsey suggests, I would encourage you to study the people you want to be like and imitate their daily habits. Imitate those who are living a good, quality life and living into their nineties and beyond. Most people who are living great quality lives are engaging in very common activities in their everyday living. These people are spending time with people they love and care about daily, taking naps or taking time for self-care, and most importantly, eating lots of fruits and vegetables.

This newer phenomenon that you have to eat all the time throughout the day is recent and barely has any truth to it.

Before technology and this life of instant gratification, humans were living and thriving on a hunting and gathering life. This means that for centuries, people ate according to nature, there were periods of time where people were not eating and went through periods of fasting because there was no food available. During periods where there was no food consumption, the body actually had time to heal and rejuvenate. Whereas we no longer get this period of fasting and rejuvenation because we are constantly eating, and instead of having our body focus on healing, our body is always having to focus on digestion. We have even been misinformed to believe that if we do not eat continuously throughout the day our metabolism will slow down, and we will continue to gain weight. You will learn in a later section about fasting that, in fact, the opposite is true.

Nature's Good in Your Grocery Store

Let me take you on a quick store tour. This is going to be a totally new experience for you. You have been so used to eating processed food and premade food. You are probably used to walking up and down those long aisles in the grocery store. It's actually not that complicated because most of the aisles in the grocery stores should not be included in your meals. Most of the food that you will find that are good and nutritious for you will be found right in the produce department, with a very few exceptions in the frozen and dairy departments. Frozen foods and dairy should be eaten sparingly, only in emergency cases where life gets busier than usual. Most fruits and vegetables in the produce department are pretty much unlimited. There are a variety of foods in the produce department. I would encourage you to try out a variety of colors. Each color gives your body a chance to absorb different vitamins and minerals.

Even though you can eat as many fruits and vegetables as you want, not all fruits and vegetables are created equally, and some may not be good for you to consume. Use your best judgment to buy the most nutritious food to fuel your body. If ever in doubt, anything grown from the ground that came from God as part of nature is much better for you than anything that is chemically processed and artificially made.

You should be aware of non-organic and genetically modified (GMO) food sources. GMO foods are commonly found in the produce department. Genetically modified foods are food crops that are altered in a way that do not occur naturally. Genetically modified foods are not required to be labeled. Anything that is not labeled non-GMO or USDA organic has the potential to be genetically modified. According to the American Academy of Environmental Medicine (AAEM), studies in animals have shown that GMO foods cause serious health risks, such as infertility, immune dysregulation, and intestinal damage. Several animal studies have also confirmed an association between GMO foods and diseases. The AAEM even goes as far as to recommend physicians educate their patients to avoid eating GMO foods and to consider the role that GMO foods can play in the development of diseases. Eleven crops from GMO seed are available commercially in the United States. They are sugar beets, canola, soy, cotton, corn, zucchini, yellow summer squash, potatoes, alfalfa, papaya, and apples. Any fresh or packaged foods containing these ingredients may possibly be genetically modified.

The best foods to fuel your body with are those that are in season, organic, local, and fresh. However, they tend to come at a higher cost, especially when a particular food you like is out of season, such as blueberries and strawberries. But each and every healthy food is absolutely worth your money. I get that organic and non-GMO foods can get too pricey. The best way to work around this is to use aluminum-free baking soda to wash your produce if you can't buy organic. This will be the best way to get rid of all the wax and pesticide on your produce. You want to use one to two teaspoon of aluminum-free baking soda in one liter of water. Let it soak for ten to fifteen minutes and rinse it off with water.

The frozen section is reserved for only frozen fruits and vegetables when you absolutely cannot cook fresh food. I know that life gets busy and sometimes it just works out better to reheat frozen vegetables. Be cautious not to use the microwave to reheat any of your food. Microwave causes radiation to the body and changes the form of food that causes a variety of health issues. The best way to reheat your food is to steam or boil your vegetables on the stove or bake it in the oven.

The only food in the dairy department that is acceptable to fuel your body with is eggs. Not all eggs are fair game. It is best to purchase eggs that are both organic and free range. If you must choose between organic, cage-free, or free-range eggs, choose organic. Organic eggs must have an organic feed without animal byproduct. They must have some access to the outdoors, and in most cases, except for illnesses, antibiotics cannot be used. Free-range and cage-free have no limitation to antibiotic use. Free range chickens have access to the outdoors and even though their daily feed is not organic, they at least get the chance to eat grass and insects that are outdoors. Cage-free eggs are not required to get any outdoor access and the feed is also not organic.

Yogurts that can be found in the dairy department, which have been perceived as healthy, are usually filled with too much sugar and have gone through too much processing, changing the health benefits that yogurt claims to have. If you must have yogurt, homemade yogurt is super easy to make, which I will include in the resource section (see Appendix C). The disadvantages of cow's milk have the same disadvantages as yogurts. It is best to drink plant-based milk, such as almond milk.

Don't forget to include healthy fats in each of your meals. Healthy fats give us the benefits we need to support our healthy lifestyle. They provide us with energy, reduce cravings, and make us feel fuller longer. Include fats, such as avocados, olive oil, and coconut oil. Nuts and seeds are great sources of fat for the body, such as cashews, almond, walnuts, and pistachios. As much as possible, try avoiding peanuts, they tend to get a bit moldy.

With natural sweeteners—if you must use sweeteners—please stick with honey. Honey is made from nature and although it should still be limited, it is the best choice if you need a sweetener. Another awesome tasting natural sweetener is dates. Dates can be added to your recipes as an alternative to sugar.

Spice your life and food up by adding natural herbs and spices to your meals, such as rosemary, dill weed, basil, and nutmeg. Both dried and fresh are great for your health.

Make sure you are making your own salad dressing. It doesn't have to be hard or complicated. Olive oil is a great base for salad dressing (see Appendix D for recipes and ideas).

Of course, my favorite topic is your source of meat and protein. Avoid all processed and deli meat. Eat seafoods that are high in omega-3 oils, such as salmon, shrimp, crab, lobster, and clams. Organic chicken. Organic grass-fed beef. If possible, eat beef that has the bone in it. Making beef and chicken broth is great for healing your gut, as it draws out the gelatin, connective tissues, and minerals out of the bone. And better yet, you know what the best source of protein is? I am sure you probably never heard of it or even tried it, but it's the organs of the animal. Yep, you guessed it! It's the liver, heart, brain, gizzard, and kidneys that are filled with the most nutrition. Eating animal organs is probably a totally different concept for you. Don't worry. I am going to show exactly how you can enjoy animal organs without completely changing your entire meals. Yes, believe it or not, you can add animal organs right into your bunless burger (see Appendix E for animal organ recipes).

Stick to tea and water as your source of liquid.

Don't get too overwhelmed. Just trust how your body is feeling and trust that God will always provide you with naturally good food.

Great Digestive Health Means Great Health

"All disease begins in the gut."
– Hippocrates

We are discovering more and more about how important the digestive tract is in our everyday health. Did you know that the amount of bacteria in our gut alone is more than all the cells in our entire body? Our digestive tracts need both good and bad bacteria to operate effectively. However, the ideal gut should comprise of more good bacteria than bad bacteria. Even more importantly, did you know that seventy to eighty percent of our immune system lies in our digestive tract? Our immune system is responsible for fighting off disease and viruses in our bodies. The importance of our digestive health is exactly why I want to take some time to focus on how you can improve your digestion. Improving your gut health improves both your overall health and will also help reduce your cravings.

Our digestion is also known as our second brain. As previously mentioned, this means that the condition of our gut has the potential to affect how we feel. This means that our gut exists to do more than just digest your food and absorb the nutrients from the food you eat. If you are lacking the nutrition, vitamins, and minerals your digestive tract needs to thrive, your emotions will also suffer. As soon as your digestive tract is healthy and working properly, your moods and emotions will become stable and you will feel better. A healthy digestive tract will keep you focused and increase your energy.

Eating the right food to support our digestive system is extremely important in order to prevent leaky gut. Leaky gut develops over a period of time, when the processed and unhealthy food we eat gets into our digestive tract. The toxins and bad bacteria that come along with our processed foods pass through our intestinal walls and into our bloodstream. Once it is in our blood, our body's defense system will think the body is being attacked by invaders and will start to attack our own bodies. This will cause a cascade of other health diseases and concerns, including bloating, stomach pains, fatigue, and even food sensitivities.

Some of the easiest and most important steps you can implement into your everyday life to improve your digestive tract and immune system are:

- Eat fresh vegetables and fruits which will give you all the fibers and nutrients your gut and body craves and needs.
- Drinking water will help you detox and help keep your bowel movements moving so that you do not keep those bad bacteria sitting in your digestive tract too long.
- Eat fermented foods that are supportive of your gut health. Raw, unprocessed, fermented food is best. Fermented foods contain good bacteria that can help the digestive tract operate properly. Fermented foods include sauerkraut, kimchi, kefir, and kombucha. Believe it or not, you can ferment a variety of fruits

and vegetables. You can always make yourself some homemade fermented food, if you cannot find any raw unprocessed fermented food in your local grocery store (see Appendix F for fermented food recipes).

- Drink bone broth daily. You can either drink bone broth like you do tea, or you can choose to make a soup out of your bone broth. You can use either organic chicken with the bone in it or organic grass-fed beef with bone to make your bone broth. Bone broth is extremely good for our health. It is dense in nutrients, like amino acids and vitamins. It contains nutrients that we search for in forms of supplemental tablets, such as collagen; which promises to keep us looking young, reduces joint and knee pain, and promotes a healthy heart (see Appendix G for bone broth recipes).

- Invest in a good quality probiotic supplement that will help support your gut. Pay attention to the bottle and its label. Look for brands that include live bacteria, billions of organisms, which means it should at least include five to one-hundred billion colony-forming units. Make sure it has multiple strands, and make sure your supplement does not have any fillers, only pure ingredients.

- Avoid antibiotics at all cost. We are so used to depending on antibiotics that we have forgotten just how much of an inconvenience it really is. Antibiotics kill all bacteria, good and bad, which will require months if not years of working hard to build up an optimal and healthy gut.

Restricted Eating for Healing

I want to introduce you to intermittent fasting for healing. I am sure you have heard of the good and the bad myths regarding intermittent fasting. I believe intermittent fasting and its benefits outweigh some of the perceptions our culture has about it. Intermittent fasting is not starving, it is merely withholding food for a period of time to allow the body to take a break so that healing and detoxification can happen in the body. When we consume food, up to eighty percent of our daily energy may be used to digest food. With so much of our energy constantly used to process the food we eat, the energy that is left from our energy source is not sufficient enough to heal and regenerate our bodies.

Our food is our energy source. When our bodies are no longer getting energy through our food source, it is only than that our body can start using our stored fat as energy. When we are constantly eating and not giving our body enough time to use up our stored fat, we gain weight. In order to restore balance to our bodies, we need to extend the amount of time that we are not eating so that we can burn more fat and energy.

My recommendation for starting your journey on intermittent fasting is to listen to your body. There are twenty-four hours in a day. I found it challenging but not impossible when I started with an eating window of eight hours, and allowing my body to fast and rest for sixteen hours each day. During my eight-hour eating window, I was able to include breakfast, lunch, and dinner as needed. Eventually, as I got used to intermittent fasting, there were days I decided I was only hungry for two or even just one meal a day. I would recommend you limit your snacking in between meals; the less your body has to focus on digesting food, the better. The more you feel comfortable with fasting, the more you can increase your hours of fasting. I would not recommend increasing your fasting window too quickly. Take at least one month to allow your body to adapt to your current fasting window before increasing your fasting window. For example, the first month would be fasting for sixteen hours every twenty-four hours, the second month will be fasting for seventeen hours, and the third month would be fasting for eighteen hours. Take it slow and steady.

The benefits of fasting include, but are definitely not limited to:

- Weight loss
- Reducing insulin resistance and better control of diabetes
- Improving brain function and focus
- Improving immune system
- Reducing inflammation
- Preventing illnesses and diseases

Discover Your Zest for Physical Activity

Physical activity is a must in your new binge-free lifestyle. It's going to keep you busy and away from food. It's going to make you feel great. It's going to allow you to get in shape and get healthy. Physical activity does not have to be rigorous or boring. It might be a bit intimidating at first, but trust me, you will get the hang of it.

You need to experiment and find something you love and something that will not make you feel like giving up. Pay attention to yourself and no one else. Remember why you are there in the first place. If you are taking a class, except for the instructor, everyone else is too busy paying attention to themselves, chances are they are not even looking at you.

If you are anything like me, I used to hate going to the gym or getting myself involved in any physical activity, but that was only because I was not yet able to find something I love. I found my passion for physical activity when I found Zumba at my local gym. I am also warning you that it is important to know that the instructor and her style of teaching makes a huge difference in finding a physical activity you love. My first three Zumba classes were with different instructors that just did not fit my goals, dancing style, or activity level. It was finally during my fourth Zumba class that I found the instructor I loved. You better bet I kept going back for more!

Zumba is where I found my zest for physical activity, and it has given me the courage to try other physical activity that I might be able and willing to add to my current physical routine.

I even tried pole dancing as an exercise and I love it! Even more recently, I gave aerial silks a try. It isn't for me, but I do not regret trying it. It was totally worth the experiment.

Find something you love and keep moving!

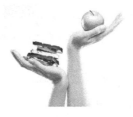

Chapter 8

The Obstacles

*Y*ay! You made it! By now, you should feel differently and should have started creating a new lifestyle for yourself. Even though this book should be easy to comprehend, easy to follow, and easy to implement, there will definitely be some things that may come up, and you may feel like you need a little more support.

Remember, we are all different and unique. Even if you follow these techniques exactly as presented or exactly as my clients did, you are expected to yield slightly different results and outcomes. While implementing these techniques, things that are specifically related to you may come up. Depending on your situation, you might find yourself needing a little bit more support or adjustment. Your nutritional protocol might need a little adjustment based on your needs or preferences. You may come to find that you may need a little more support on detox symptoms that start to show up as you detox your mind, body, and emotions.

As you are going through some of the chapters, new emotions may show up in your life. Specifically I found this occurring in the chapter of exploring your emotions, as you are releasing your old negative emotions. You may need more support in understanding how to either embrace these new positive emotions or understand how and when it is best to continue to release negative emotions that seem to still be trapped. Sometimes, taking time to feel your emotions is just downright emotional, and you might need someone who will walk you through each step, hold your hand, and tell you that everything will be perfectly fine.

You might also find yourself just needing more support than the book can give you. Who doesn't want a personal health coach or personal human contact? We all do. We all need that one person who can hold you accountable, or that one person who can keep you moving forward by motivating you so that you don't give up like you have done too many times in the past. Someone to keep you from being too tough on yourself and end up beating yourself up. Someone to stop your self-doubt right in the middle of its tracks. This is where I can come in and become your cheerleader cheering you on, or water boy handing to you all the resources you will need to succeed.

Finding Yourself a Best Friend

In the middle of my health coaching sessions with clients, I can hear the negative talk and the self-doubt that these clients think about. I just can't imagine what actually goes on in their mind, if they are already verbally expressing to me these self-doubts and are constantly beating themselves up.

I had one particular client, Franni, that came to me. She was shy and reserved and came to me frustrated and feeling emotionally unstable. I often heard her talking herself out of the process and out of living a healthier lifestyle. She often talked negatively about herself in front of me. She had so much self-doubt. She thought it was impossible to implement a lot of the things I educated her on, and even if she did implement them, she wondered if they would work.

I knew I had to intervene. This much self-doubt and negativity would never lead her to the healthier lifestyle she always wanted. I walked Franni through an exercise to help her understand the effects of beating one's self up and self-doubt. I had Franni take ten minutes to write down all the daily things she tells herself, including any self-doubt, self-talk, belief, and self-criticism. I asked her to pretend that I was her best friend who she sees on a regular basis. I read back to her everything she wrote down. After reading back to her everything she wrote, I asked her, if her best friend talked to her like she talks to herself, would she remain best friends with this person? She knew where I was going with this, and that was when emotions and pain started flowing out of her. She admitted that there was no way she would stick with such a friend. She also had to question herself why she would allow such horrible self-talk and self-criticism day in and day out. At this point, she was very emotional, but to get my point across, I had to dig deeper in order to give her a better understanding of the pain and destruction she was actually causing herself. I continue to ask her if she thought these thoughts and words were of God's or not. In this one session, she discovered why she has been feeling so depressed. She realized that anyone who talked to themselves the way she did would have no choice but to be depressed. She now had a better understanding of my previous explanation about how negative emotions can affect a person's health and the importance of releasing these trapped negative emotions right away.

You Are So Awesomely Unique

By now I hope you know how awesomely unique and special you truly are; both you and your life experiences are what makes you awesome. Similar to many of my clients, I had to learn that my uniqueness allowed me to be who I am today and who I want to become in my future. My unique situations and challenges I faced daily were exactly why it only made sense to me to further leverage myself by investing more time, effort, and energy in me. For my clients and I, this meant investing in someone who could hold my hand through my specific experiences and situations because I couldn't possibly know all I needed to know to get through my own unique situations and challenges.

I want you to take a moment to just imagine how support beyond the techniques and concepts this book provides looks and feels to you. Everyone's support systems look a little bit different when creating the life you want. I had a client, Denise, that came to me looking for support in her home. With a five-month-old daughter and a husband that worked forty hours plus each week, she wasn't sure how to build a home that would be supportive of her new healthy lifestyle. We both had to sit down and take some time to write down her weekly schedule so that her husband was on the same page, and so that he could try to work around her schedule. We wrote down a schedule for when she would need time in her daily schedule to meditate, spend time with God, and if needed, release some emotions. We even wrote down her once weekly meal planning sessions so that her husband could be sure that he was home to watch the baby while she took some time to meal prep for the week and not fall back into her binge eating cycles. Just imagine how much easier this journey would be for you if you could implement the right support system for yourself. Don't hesitate to ask me how I can help. Let me know how I can be of service to you. How can I help you personally leverage yourself above and beyond living a binge-free life?

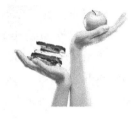

Chapter 9

Marching Orders

Solid Understanding, Solid Foundation

I am so excited that you have come this far. This tells me that you are serious about taking control of your own health and binge eating habits. I am glad that you have learned all you need to know in order to free yourself from binge eating for good. Keep in mind, it's not just about knowing what you need to know, but most importantly, it's about doing what you need to do to reach your goals.

By now, you should have a solid understanding of how you can use all the concepts and techniques in this book to support yourself and set yourself free from binge eating—not only focusing on the nutritional aspect, but on yourself as a whole person with a mind, body, and spirit. You should now understand how much of an impact and difference it makes when you have all the right support system and techniques in place in order to successfully tackle binge eating, with less frustration and stress.

Quantum physics has taught us how we are connected to the energy around us and how you can use this knowledge to manifest the reality you want. You have learned that building a relationship with the Lord and faithfully relying on Him will help you renew your mind and turn away from all your unhealthy thoughts and negative perspectives on food. You now understand how negative emotions can affect you and how important it is to take the time to process those negative emotions and quickly release them. Furthermore, this far you have been brave enough to have taken all the knowledge you gained about quantum physics, the Lord, and emotions to create environments that are supportive to your journey of freeing yourself from binge eating.

My Wish for You

My wish for you is that you find healing, not just for your physical body, but also for your spiritual, mental, and emotional health. There are many layers to healing, a lifetime full of healing, I encourage you to continue to dig deeper as you manifest more healing into your life. I hope this healing will bring you stability and peace. I hope that once you can control your binge eating cycle, that you will find the zest and motivation you once had for life and work.

Most of all, my wish for you is for you to continue to use the daily routine you have learned to create for yourself because these daily habits can create for you an even brighter future beyond getting rid of your binge eating habit. You can use these exact concepts and techniques to create anything and everything you want for your future. The only thing that can limit you is your own imagination and self-doubt.

I hope that you find your own story and testimony in this journey so that you can bless others with your story. In a world that seems to have a healthcare system that just isn't working, there are many people looking for your help, and looking to be inspired by you. Be the inspiration that makes a difference!

So, what's next?! Stay in touch, of course!

I have created a Facebook group exclusively for individuals who have purchased this book. In this group, you can expect to receive support not only from me, but also your peers. This page was created so that you can have a respectful place to share your experiences, ask questions, and simply to encourage and motivate each other. I also created this page so that you can continue to stay connected to me as I share with you some valuable information and keep you motivated and moving in the right direction. Click here to visit us on our Facebook page.

If you are looking for further resources and support to help you on your journey, please visit me at

www.lindamovement.com.

I read any and all emails.

I get easily excited about all the emails I get from my clients and everyone this book has touched. I read and reply to each and every email personally. I hope you stay in touch and send me an email. Even if it's just an email to say, "Hi." However, I love emails that let me know how you are doing, and how this book has impacted you. Your emails let me know the difference I am making, and I love that!

It's easy to send me an email. I can be reached at linda@ lindamovement.com.

Good luck and I hope to hear from you soon!

References

Dispenza, Dr. Joe. (2012). Breaking the Habit of Being Yourself: How to Lose Your Mind and Create a New One (1st ed.). Hay House, Inc.

Nelson, Dr. Bradley. (2007). The Emotion Code (1st ed.). Mesquite, NV: Wellness Unmasked Publishing.

Lipton, Ph. D., Bruce H. (2015). The Biology of Belief. Hay House, Inc.

Pert, Ph. D., Candace B. (1997). Molecules of Emotions. New York, New York: Touchstone.

Meyer, Joyce. (2018). Healing the Soul of a Woman. New York, New York: Hachette Book Group, Inc.

https://academic.oup.com/ptj/article/81/8/1455/2857674

https://insights.ovid.com/crossref? an=00000658-201102000-00009

https://www.mayoclinic.org/diseases-conditions/insomnia/expert-answers/lack-of-sleep/faq-20057757

https://www.ncbi.nlm.nih.gov/pmc/articles/PMC3894660/

https://charliefoundation.org/diet-plans/

https://www.cdc.gov/diabetes/statistics/slides/long_term_trends.pdf

https://www.washingtonpost.com/news/wonk/wp/2014/09/16/the-decline-of-the-small-american-family-farm-in-one-chart/? noredirect=on&utm_term=.4ec8b43724aa

https://www.newsmax.com/fastfeatures/gmos-health-foods-genetic-engineering/2015/02/09/id/622630/

https://delishably.com/dairy/Organic-Eggs-vs-Free-Range-and-Cage-Free-Alternatives

https://delishably.com/dairy/Organic-Eggs-vs-Free-Range-and-Cage-Free-Alternatives

https://draxe.com/birth-control-pills/

https://www.ncbi.nlm.nih.gov/pmc/articles/PMC4394736/

https://www.ncbi.nlm.nih.gov/pmc/articles/PMC1456909/

http://www.businessdictionary.com/definition/leverage.html

https://www.aaemonline.org/gmo.php

https://www.mindbodygreen.com/articles/probiotics-how-to-choose-the-right-one-tell-if-theyre-high-quality-and-more

Appendix A

My Daily Schedule

MY DAILY SCHEDULE

7:00 AM

Alarm goes off and it's time to get ready for the day.

7:10 AM

I am up to brush my teeth and wash my face.

7:30 AM

I am in my office ready to start my morning rountine. My morning routine consists of a quick stretch, mediation, some time with God, and releasing negative emotions, as needed.

8:30 AM

I cook my lunch for the day and pack it to go.

9:00 AM

I get ready and am out the door for work.

11:00 AM

Lunchtime is around the corner. I start to think about food. Once in awhile I'll crave junk food and I must take some time to revert my mind back to the healthy food I packed.

12:00 PM

It is lunch time and it has been a stressful morning at work. Before I eat my lunch, I take a few minutes to evaluate whether I'm actually hungry or just emotionally/spiritually starving.

4:00 PM

I start to mentally go over what I am cooking for dinner tonight.

6:15 PM

Enjoying dinner with my husband.

7:00 PM

Take a break for some "me" time.

8:15 PM

My evening sweet tooth tells me I'm craving for something sweet. I put on some upbeat music and head to the gym instead of eating sweets.

9:00 PM

I take some time to relax and wind down for the night and mentally prepare for tomorrow.

Negative Emotions Chart
(Releasing Your Trapped Emotions)

Negative Emotions Chart		
Column A	Column B	Column C
Row 1 Abandoned	Empty	Mocked
Abused	Envious	Nervous
Anger	Exposed	Powerless
Anxiety	Failure	Pride
Ashamed	Fearful	Rejected
Row 2 Attacked	Frustrated	Resentment
Betrayed	Grief	Sadness
Bitter	Guilty	Shameful
Blame	Harrassed	Terror
Broken-Hearted	Hated	Trapped
Row 3 Burdened	Helpless	Vulnerable
Condemned	Hopelessness	Undersirable
Conflicted	Humiliated	Worthless
Criticized	Hurt	Worry
Decieved	Insulted	Trapped
Row 4 Depressed	Intimdated	Violated
Desperate	Insecure	Vulnerable
Disappointed	Isolated	Undersirable
Disgust	Manipulated	Used
Embarassed	Mistreated	Worthless

Appendix C

Recipe for Homemade Yogurt

Homemade Yogurt

Ingredients List:
- -1 14-15 oz. full-fat organic coconut milk
- -2 teaspoons gelatin
- -2-3 capsules probiotic
- -Honey (as needed, optional)
- -Fruits (as needed, optional)

Directions:
1. Pour the organic coconut milk into a glass jar big enough to fit all the coconut milk.
2. Twist open the probiotic capsules and dump them into the coconut milk.
3. Stir the probiotic thoroughly into the organic coconut milk.
4. Cover the glass jar with a cheesecloth and secure it with a rubber band

5. Set the jar aside in a warm spot away from direct light for 24–48 hours.

6. Let the magic happen—fermentation takes place (so that you can get all those good bacteria into your digestive tract!).

7. Once the yogurt is thick enough for your preference, place it in the refrigerator for another 8–12 hours so that it can continue to thicken.

8. After 8–12 hours in the refrigerator you are ready to eat the yogurt.

9. For better taste, feel free to add some raw organic unprocessed honey and your choice of fruits.

Recipe for Homemade Salad Dressing

Olive Oil Zest Salad Dressing

Ingredients List (remember you can easily adjust salad dressing ingredients to your own preference):
- -2–3 tablespoons olive oil
- -1 lemon juice
- -Dash of salt (or to taste)
- -Dash of black pepper (or to taste)
- -1 teaspoon honey

Directions:
1. Squeeze lemon juice into a bowl.
2. Mix the rest of the ingredients together into the lemon juice thoroughly.
3. Enjoy! Use as much as needed for dressing your salad.

Avocado Lemon Salad Dressing

Ingredients List:
- -2 tablespoons olive oil
- -1 lemon juice
- -1 ripe avocado
- -Dash of salt (or to taste)
- -Dash of black pepper (or to taste)
- -1 bunch cilantro
- -1 clove garlic

Directions:
1. Peel the avocado and scoop it into the blender.
2. Squeeze the lemon juice into the blender.
3. Add all other ingredients into the blender and blend thoroughly.
4. Enjoy! Use as much as needed for dressing your salad.

Appendix E

Animal Organ Recipe

Beef Patties

Ingredients List:
- -2 pounds lean ground organic grass-fed beef
- -1/2 pound liver (you can use organic chicken, beef, or lamb liver)
- -1 teaspoon garlic powder
- -1 teaspoon onion powder
- -1/2 teaspoon salt (or salt to taste)
- -Dash of black pepper (or to taste)
- -1 egg

Directions:
1. Pulse liver mixture in food processor until coarsely puréed.
2. In a bowl mix the liver, ground beef and all the seasoning until well combined.
3. Form the mixture into disc-shaped patties.

4. Cook the patties in a pan on medium-high for about 5-7 minutes on each side.
5. Enjoy your organ mixed patties with other veggies, like lettuce, tomatoes, onions!

Heart Stir-fry (Another one of my mother's homemade dishes.)

Ingredients List:
- -1-2 pounds heart (you can use organic chicken, beef, or lamb heart)
- -1/2 teaspoon salt (or salt to taste)
- -Dash of black pepper (or to taste)
- -3-4 onion scallions
- -1/4 cilantro bunch
- -1 tablespoon of coconut oil

Directions:
1. Slice the heart into thin slices of meat.
2. Put the coconut oil into a pan and cook the thin slices of heart. (If you are new to organ meat, treat this whole process of slicing and cooking exactly like you would beef or chicken)
3. Add your salt and pepper while cooking the heart.
4. Once the meat is fully cooked, turn off the stove, and mix in your onion and cilantro.
5. Enjoy! You can eat this with other side dishes or vegetables, like you would any other stir-fry dish.

Fermented Food Recipe

Kimchi

Ingredients List:

- -1 head napa cabbage
- -1/4 cup sea salt or Himalayan Pink salt
- -1 teaspoon freshly grated ginger
- -5 cloves grated garlic
- -3 tablespoons Korean red pepper flakes (gochugaru)
- -1 daikon radish
- -3 carrots
- -3 scallions
- -6 cups of water (or enough to soak the cabbage)

Directions:

1. Cut the napa cabbage laterally into about 2–inch pieces. Place these cut up pieces of cabbage into a bowl big enough for the cabbage and 6 cups of water.
2. Dissolve the salt into 2 cups of lukewarm water to make the brine.

3. Pour your brine over the cabbage; add the rest of the remaining 4 cups of water. Let the cabbage soak in the brine for at least 2–4 hours. Make sure the cabbage is completely submerged in the water. You may need something heavy to hold the cabbage down.

4. While you cabbage is soaking dice the daikon radish, carrots and scallions into sticks.

5. You will also want to make the paste for the kimchi. Stir together in a small bowl the garlic, ginger, red pepper flakes, and honey. Stir until you have a smooth paste.

6. Mix the paste with the daikon radish, carrots, and scallions thoroughly.

7. After soaking the cabbage, drain the cabbage reserving about 1 cup of the brine for later use. Rinse the cabbage under cold water and wait 15 minutes for all the water out to drain out. Repeat this step two more times to ensure all the salt is rinsed off.

8. Place the cabbage back in a large bowl. Mix the scallions, apple/onion mixture and paste into the cabbage. Mix well to coat all pieces.

9. Place the kimchi into an airtight glass jar or mason jar. Pack down the vegetables the best you can, leave at least one inch from the top of the jar for air or gas. Use the brine you saved earlier, if needed to cover vegetables.

10. With the jar close, let it sit in room temperature for 2–5 day. Check on the kimchi once a day to ensure all vegetables are submerged, if not use a spoon to push the vegetables down. When the kimchi taste as desired, store the kimchi in the refrigerator.

11. Enjoy!

Pickles (or any vegetable you prefer. This is a simple recipe that you can use to ferment a variety of vegetables.)

Ingredients List:

- -5 cucumbers (or any vegetables you prefer, including radish, carrots, zucchini, green beans, broccoli, cauliflower, garlic, jalapenos, or asparagus)
- -2 tablespoons sea salt or Himalayan Pink salt
- -1 teaspoon honey
- -3–4 cloves garlic
- -1 bunch dill
- -Filtered water (enough to submerge all of the cucumbers)
- -A pinch red pepper flakes (optional)

Directions:

1. Clean your cucumbers.
2. Slice the cucumbers in to strips that are about ¼ inch-thick, and long enough to leave about 2 inches of room from the top of the jar.
3. Pressed down as much of the cucumbers as you can into a mason jar. Leave about 2 inches of headspace.
4. Add your garlic clove, dill, and red pepper flakes into the jar of cucumbers.
5. Prepare your brine in small bowl by dissolving the salt and honey into about 1 cup of water.
6. Pour the brine into the mason jar.
7. Add more water as needed to the jar. Make sure to leave at least 1–2 inches of headspace.

8. Leave the vegetables out at room temperature to ferment.

9. Open the mason jar once a day to check on the cucumbers. Continue to push down the cucumber under the water.

10. The fermented process should be completed in about 4–5 days or to taste. Refrigerate when ready. Your pickles should taste firm and crisp.

Recipe for Bone Broth

Beef Bone Broth
(This is actually the simple but delicious ingredients my mother used to make her version of the best tasting homemade beef bone broth. You can choose to cook your bone broth in a slow cooker or you can choose to boil it on your stove.)

Ingredients List:
- -2–4 pounds mixed organic grass-fed beef bones (include a mix of oxtail, shank, marrow bones, or short-ribs)
- -1–2 teaspoons gelatin (optional—my favorite brand is Great Lakes)
- -2–3 stalks lemon grass
- -1 handful thinly sliced ginger root
- -3–6 quarters filtered water (need to at least cover up all the bones)
- -1 teaspoon salt (or salt to taste)
- -Dash of black pepper (or to taste)

Directions:

1. Clean and rinse the beef off well.
2. Fill your stainless-steel pot or slow cooker up with water.
3. Place the beef in the pot/slow cooker.
4. Place all other ingredients into the pot/slower cooker.
5. Cover the pot/slower cooker.
   - When boiling your bones on the stove: Bring the bones to a boil or simmer over high heat. Once the bones are boiling, continue to cover the pot and turn the temperature down as low as possible and let the bones cook at a low simmer for at least 18–48 hours.
   - When cooking with a slow cooker: Cook your bone on low for about 18–48 hours.
6. Occasionally check the pot/slower cooker for the foam on the surface of the pot. Skim off the foam and continue to add water to make sure the bone is covered for the first 1–2 hours.
7. Once the bone broth is ready you can choose to strain the broth with a cheesecloth or a strainer to remove all the bits of bones and vegetables.
8. Let the bone broth cool and transfer it to a airtight jar and freeze or refrigerate the broth for future use.

Chicken Bone Broth (This is actually the simple but delicious ingredients my mother used to make her version of the best tasting homemade beef bone broth.)

Ingredients List:
- -1 whole organic chicken (with the feet, if at all possible, the feet are the best source of gelatin)
- -1–2 teaspoons gelatin (optional—my favorite brand is Great Lakes)
- -2–3 stalks lemon grass
- -3–4 quarters filtered clean water (need to at least cover up the whole chicken)
- -1 teaspoon salt (or salt to taste)
- -Dash of black pepper (or to taste)

Directions:
1. Clean and rinse the chicken. It is optional to cut the chicken up into smaller pieces or you can choose to boil the whole chicken (I prefer to cut my chicken into smaller pieces).
2. Fill your stainless-steel pot or slow cooker up with water.
3. Place the chicken in the pot/slow cooker.
4. Place all other ingredients into the pot/slower cooker.
5. Cover the pot/slower cooker.
   - When boiling your bones on the stove: Bring the chicken to a boil or simmer over high heat. Once the chicken is boiling, continue to cover the pot and turn the temperature down as low as possible

and let the chicken cook at a low simmer for at least 18–48 hours.

- When cooking with a slow cooker: Cook your chicken on low for about 18–48 hours.

6. Occasionally check the pot/slower cooker for the foam on the surface of the pot. Skim off the foam and continue to add water to make sure the bone is covered for the first 1–2 hours.

7. Once the chicken is ready you can choose to strain the broth with a cheesecloth or a strainer to remove all the bits of bones and vegetables.

8. Let the bone broth cool and transfer it to an airtight jar and freeze or refrigerate the broth for future use.

About the Author

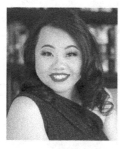 Linda Vang was tired of being stuck in the rut of her own never-ending binge eating cycles. After receiving her health coaching certificate, even though she knew all she needed to know nutritionally to stop binge eating, she was still left feeling stuck in the same cycle. She continued her education through a training program for holistic practitioners and received additional training that gave her knowledge on how to best support her whole being, including her mind, body, and spirit. She is committed to educating women on how to

take care of themselves in the midst of our busy lives and to live out their best life with energy and passion.

Linda lives in Minnesota with her husband and enjoys evening walks with him. She is lively and turns it up a notch when there is music. She also enjoys her favorite activities of Zumba, karaoke, and pole dancing for fitness. Linda believes in enjoying life to the fullest and is a major advocate for building an enjoyable work-life balance after working in the human resources field for ten-plus years, before dedicating her life as a health coach.

Thank You!

Here's a Gift for You!

I want to take some time to thank you for purchasing my book. This book purchase means so much to me. I love that each purchase means that I can invest more into creating a movement that can change the lives and health of each person I touch. As a thank you, I am gifting you a three-part video series to help you gear up for a successful journey to conquer your binge eating and beyond.

Now that you know everything you need to know to successfully control your binge eating habit, I want you to know how important it is to actually continue to implement these techniques into your daily lives. In order for you to stay motivated and keep moving forward in your progress so far, I have created a three-part series that I feel strongly about. This video series is short, but powerful. Each video will include an impactful action step to take that will help you gear up to create a life you love and a life that you can enjoy for years to come. These activities will help you realize how important your health really is, and how important it is to keep moving towards your goals. What are you waiting for?! Go to lindamovement.com to get started today!

CPSIA information can be obtained
at www.ICGtesting.com
Printed in the USA
JSHW031423101220
10133JS00011B/42